Ketogenic Diet

Table Of Contents

Introduction

This book contains proven steps and strategies on how to effectively prepare delicious, low-carb, and high-fat meals that will help the body transition into a lighter and leaner physique. It is expected that following a ketogenic-friendly meal plan, together with its nutritious recipes, will have a positive impact on one's longevity and quality of life.

The ketogenic diet's objective is to promote fat loss and weight management by following a healthy food ratio of high fat, moderate protein and very few carbs in our daily meals. This unique balance of carbs, protein and fat will subsequently trigger nutritional ketosis, a natural process that breaks down fat cells and turns it into energy.

In this book, the connection behind ketosis and weight loss will be explained in order to have greater appreciation for the ketogenic diet. You will likewise be able to see how a keto-adopted lifestyle affects blood sugar levels and prevents the onset of medical conditions that threaten one's health.

Moreover, the 70 recipes in this book that will help jumpstart a ketogenic lifestyle are categorized into 5 meals: breakfast, lunch, dinner, snack and dessert. Each recipe is easy to follow and uses natural yet low-carbohydrate ingredients that will satisfy your taste buds without adding extra inches on the waistline.

Thanks again for downloading this book, I hope you enjoy it!

Ketogenic Diet In A Nutshell

Every diet or eating lifestyle has its pro and cons alongside challenges that make first timers find it harder to adopt. Before we get to see what mistakes or pitfalls come with Ketogenic diet, let's first understand what the diet entails. In a nutshell, the ketogenic diet emphasizes on increasing your intake of fat and protein while reducing your intake of carbohydrates. The ketogenic diet is meant to restrict carbohydrate intake in order to control your blood sugar levels. Since our body's main source of energy is glucose, if your body is low in glucose, the body is forced to find other sources of energy to sustain the body's metabolism processes. Once under the "starvation" mode, your body is said to undergo ketosis. Simply put ketosis is a process in which the liver begins to synthesize ketone bodies and fatty acids as alternative sources of fuel. The stored fats are thereby broken down in the liver into fatty acids and other products that we now call ketone bodies. The ketone bodies are then oxidized as the main energy source to provide fuel for your body in place of carbohydrates.

The ketogenic diet was initially designed to help people suffering from epilepsy but with the availability of epileptic drugs, the diet is not as effective for those suffering from epilepsy. However, there has been a lot of success with the diet being effective in helping people lose weight. For you to lose weight with the Keto diet plan, you need to restrict your carb intake to less than 50g in a day. You should then meet your daily calorie requirement from food sources that offer high amounts of fats and lean protein to sustain metabolic processes. With that understanding of the ketogenic diet, let us now look at how you can lose weight with the ketogenic diet.

How The Ketogenic Diet works

The Ketogenic diet works by triggering a state of ketosis once your blood glucose levels are low. Ketosis is a body state in which you're at a high fat burning rate. Actually, the human brain normally runs on ketone bodies, the energy molecules found in the blood, which are processed from fat by the liver for fuel. A lower intake of carbohydrates can help trigger production of ketones bodies, and can also maintain lower levels of insulin secretion. It's important to sustain a lower insulin levels as it facilitates large amounts of ketones in the blood.

Even though low-carb intake is what is most important while on a ketogenic diet, you may at various occasions fail to achieve the maximum ketones in the blood mainly due to poor intake of proteins. And when I talk of poor protein intake it simply implies that you consume excess amounts of proteins say from fish, lean meat or seeds and nuts. The downside is that the excess protein is converted into glucose and can raise your insulin level at the expense of inhibiting ketosis. To avoid interfering with "optimal ketosis", just ensure that you eat more fat instead, as fat can induce satiety and fight cravings.

If your goal is to lose weight, you might be scared of eating a high fat diet but research has shown that healthy fatty foods like wild caught salmon, walnuts, and olive oil can actually facilitate weight loss.

Let us look at why you should adopt a ketogenic diet if you want to lose weight.

Advantages of Ketogenic Diet

Being in a state of ketosis has many benefits. If you suffer from diabetes or are pre-diabetic, obese or at the risk of developing heart disease adapting the Ketogenic diet can really help. Below are some of the benefits you get when on a low carb diet

Weight loss

Research has proven that dieters can actually lose weight while following a ketogenic diet. Actually, there have been reported cases where people have lost up to 160 pounds by switching to a ketogenic diet. A ketogenic diet serves to lower carbohydrate intake which forces your body to burn fat to produce energy. Due to the inefficiency of fat as a fuel, a lot of it has to be burned to release a relatively small amount of energy. Thus, ketosis can be very helpful in shedding that extra weight even if you are obese.

Lowers blood sugar levels

When we eat a high carb diet, the carbohydrates are broken down to glucose in the digestive tract where it is absorbed into the bloodstream. When it enters the bloodstream, it causes a spike in blood sugar and thus will force the body to produce more insulin to regulate the sugar levels. However, if you suffer from insulin resistance, your body is unable to regulate blood sugar levels and this might lead to type II diabetes. The ketogenic diet addresses this situation by lowering the amount of available glucose in the blood thus reducing the need for insulin.

Ketosis makes the body to utilize body fat for fuel

If you are on a high carbohydrate diet, the body breaks it down into glucose. The body will prefer to oxidize glucose rather than body fat since it uses less oxygen. On the other hand, ketosis makes the body efficient in burning your body fat instead so you can shed weight a lot faster. In addition, ketone bodies are very inefficient fuel and thus have very little calories relative to their mass. Therefore, if the body is in ketosis, it will burn a lot of fat in order to get adequate energy for a particular activity.

Ensures no excess fat is stored

Let's say your body has no use for excess ketones that are processed from fats, here it will simply excrete them out as urine. This is in contrast to a high carb diet where excess glucose is converted into fat and unfortunately stored "for later use". Therefore, a low carb diet does not only make it easier to lose body fat but also maintain body shape as no fat deposits are made.

Ketosis controls insulin levels

No doubt, a ketogenic diet helps lower your insulin levels to facilitate metabolism of fat into energy. Insulin has the ability to prevent the conversion of fat to energy; a process called lipolysis and a high carb diet increases the level of insulin and inhibits lipolysis. Thus, the lowered insulin levels will increase lipolysis hence more fat will be burned. In addition, the lowered insulin levels allows for the release of other beneficial hormones such as the growth hormone.

Helps burn abnormal fats

In a Ketogenic diet, majority of the fat that is burned is from the abdominal cavity what is referred to as visceral fat. As opposed to subcutaneous fat deposited under the skin, visceral fat can drive inflammation, insulin resistance and cause metabolic dysfunction. A low carb diet can help burn the visceral fat and thus can quickly get rid of that tummy fat.

While going on a ketogenic diet has many benefits, there are also downfalls to it. Let us look at some of the challenges you are likely to face while on ketosis.

Disadvantages of Ketosis

Ketosis may pose a few problems before you get used to the diet. However, you don't have to worry as most of these drawbacks are only temporary and can be corrected with time. For instance, you have to undergo a transition stage, as your body adjusts to using ketone bodies as a source of energy. Therefore, before then you may experience a number of side effects including fatigue, headaches, and nausea. Other drawbacks of the diet include:

Deficiency of micronutrients

Since foods rich in carbohydrates are restricted, you can have a deficiency of micronutrients that accompany these foods. Obviously this may lead to deficiency related conditions or diseases. However, this shouldn't worry you much as you can alternatively take vitamin and mineral supplements. Also remember to take a lot of fiber to aid in digestion, thus eat a lot of veggies.

Higher levels of cholesterol

Since the ketogenic diet requires increased intake of fats, it can cause the blood lipids to increase. This means instead of reducing cholesterol in the blood stream, the high intake of fats can cause the reverse effect of

increasing cholesterol levels. The good news is that unsaturated fatty foods like fish, nuts, seeds and beef can boost production
of the good HDL cholesterol.

Too high level of ketone bodies

There's a process referred to as Ketoacidosis in which the amount of ketone bodies multiplies and gets out of control. Such an outcome can then lead to acidosis, an effect which lowers the bloods pH, a condition that can be fatal if not treated. However, this is unlikely to affect non-diabetic people as their bodies keep blood sugar low and allow only enough ketones to be produced at any one time.

Hope by now you know how you stand to benefit by adopting the ketogenic diet and what to watch out for. In the following chapter, we are going to look at common pitfalls further and how to avoid them or recover from them.

Ketogenic Diet Pitfalls and How To Avoid Them

No doubt adopting a low-carb diet can be quite a challenge as a beginner especially if you are of the view that fat is a disaster to health and weight loss. That said; research has proven that reducing your carb intake and rather focusing on high fat and protein diet is the most efficient way to build muscle and lose weight. These two food groups have been studied to help dieters boost health and lower risks of diseases like diabetes, cancer, and cardiovascular problems.

That notwithstanding, a low-carb Ketogenic diet if implemented in a wrong manner can cause chronic inflammation, trigger hormonal imbalances and hinder weight loss. A common problem is the fact that many dieters don't differentiate between simple carbs from the complex carbs as well as how much carbohydrates they need to take to achieve ketosis as well as how their protein intake out to be. Imbalances in consumption of food groups can be addressed with prior knowledge on common pitfalls and how to avoid them. Let's see low-carb diet mistakes you should be aware of in advance:

Higher intake of carbs

By now you already know that you need to adopt a low-carb and high protein diet for weight loss but exactly what does low-carb translate to? Let's say your carb intake per day as an average American man sums up to 300 grams, reducing intake to 150 gram could be termed low-carb, right? You will be surprised that you need to go lower than that to around 20 percent of your carb calories intake! Research from American Journal of Clinical Nutrition has shown that for ketosis to take place uninterrupted, you need to maintain a carb intake of 50 grams daily.

If you live a sedentary lifestyle, 50grams intake of carbs may trigger sufficient production of ketone bodies and will cease to rely on glucose but stored fats for metabolism. The quick fix for a higher carb intake is to maintain a 50 gram intake of carbs by ensuring that you mainly consume dark-leafy green veggies. Remember that carbs don't only come from grains and processed foods but also from fruits and veggies. You need to check the carb content from fresh veggies before eating them, preferably celery, mushrooms, green beans, broccoli and lettuce. Don't be scared of eating salads often and ensure that you choose low-carb fruits and veggies. Since fruits could be rich in carbs, try selected fruits such as berries and practically avoid all grains, whether whole or processed.

Excess consumption of proteins

It's a fact that a higher intake of proteins can help boost satiety, lower cravings and actually help you get leaner as you lose weight. That said; excess intake of proteins than what your body actually requires can trigger gluconeogenesis, or the conversion of amino acids into glucose. Once this happens, the body's capability to burn fat is reduced as metabolism switches on glucose for fuel. A higher intake of 230 to 250 grams of proteins daily can hinder the body from excreting the toxic byproducts of protein metabolism such as ammonia. Furthermore, once the proteins aren't fully processed and get into the intestines, the undigested proteins undergo fermentation through the gut bacteria and yield inflammatory products. In extreme cases, protein only diet can cause loss of calcium and damage your kidneys.

So exactly how much proteins do your require? For those of you who workout, a 1.5-2.0 grams per each kilo of body weight can match well with a low-carb diet. Try to maintain protein intake to below 1.5 g/kg and ensure that the protein comes from animals and sea foods like fatty wild-caught salmon or kelp. You may also need to find out ketone concentration through a urine test even though the results might not reflect actual levels in the blood. The best way to check this out is through ketone blood test although it can be quite expensive.

Eating lesser calories from fat

The key concept of a ketogenic diet is to trigger your metabolism to burn fats rather than glucose in a bid to stop storage of fat in tissues. A lower fat intake can yield extremely low calorie intake, or cause elevated cortisol or reduced thyroid hormone functionality. What happens is when fat intake is lower than required, the production of energy is slowed down and you're unable to sustain a low-carb diet. The best way to make Ketogenic diet work is to ensure 50 percent of calories you eat come from fatty foods and oils.

The key to eating a high fat diet is to include fats at each meal, by choosing to consume fats from red-palm oil, olive oil, organic meats, fatty fish, avocados, nuts and olives. For breakfast, try the "fat coffee" trick by adding some oil, butter or heavy cream to your drink. For instance, you can add tablespoon of coconut oil and a tablespoon of butter to your morning or afternoon coffee. Blend to achieve the best consistency. The higher the fat intake, the lesser proteins and carbs you consume; which drops down insulin levels and gets you into optimal ketosis.

Also get fats by consuming fatty cuts of meat, cooked in butter if preferred, to facilitate conversion of fats and ketones for energy. Instead of just eating boneless and skinless chicken breast, try applying sufficient amounts of butter under the chicken leg skin and thigh before you cook. Use your fingers to wolf them as the butter drips your arms. Don't trim fats from your steaks but instead eat them the fatty side in. An easy way to get fats is eating bacon, and then eat it wobbly with its fat content intact.

Eating inadequate vegetables & fruit

Now that you know that even fruits and veggies have carbs, you might be tempted to eliminate all plant-based foods to maintain a 50 grams intake of carbs. However, be informed that veggies are nutrient-packed and plays a huge role in preventing diseases and curbing inflammatory reactions. Taking more veggies helps you boost your nutrients intake and reduces calories intake. You need to obtain around 5 servings daily of veggies either as a snack, main meal or a side dish. In addition to fruits and vegetables being high in nutrients, they are also high in fiber that promotes satiety and makes you eat less, thus you need them for fiber if you eliminate grains.

Ensure that you consume about 2-3 cups of carb veggies at each meal from low-glycemic carbs like green veggies, peppers, turnips, green beans, mushrooms, asparagus, egg plant, avocados, garlic and tomatoes. For fruits, ensure you limit their intake to fruits like berries to ensure you still get the important fiber and phytonutrients. A creative way to snack on fruits and veggies is to make your own salads. Also, consider healthy ingredients such as fresh herbs, balsamic vinegar, fresh lemon juice, Dijon mustard and extra-virgin olive oil for your dressing. Try this simple Soy-Ginger Dressing recipe: Whisk together 2 tablespoons of low-sodium soy sauce, minced garlic clove, 1½ teaspoon grated ginger and 2 tablespoons red wine vinegar. Then whisk the mixture into a ¼ cup of canola oil. The recommended serving size is 2 tablespoons per serving, with lesser amounts for creamier options. Try other ingredients like clove of garlic, roughly chopped scallions, mayonnaise, a medium avocado, fresh lemon juice, chopped fresh tarragon, chopped fresh parsley and chopped fresh basil. These can be blended to smoothness and then seasoned with freshly ground pepper and sea salt to taste.

Low intake of indigestible fiber

Research has shown that eating more animal proteins may cause you to eat less fiber particularly from fruits and veggies. It is important to note that dietary fiber doesn't raise your blood sugar level as it slows down glucose absorption into the blood. Fiber also makes you feel fuller for longer and fights cravings. A rule of the thumb is to consume 2-7 grams of fiber daily. Therefore, increase your fiber intake by 2-4 grams daily from consumption of veggies and fruits. Get soluble fiber from foods such as grapes, kiwi, pomegranates, blackberries, raspberries, tart cherries and blueberries. Low glycemic and fiber-rich veggies that should form your best choice include artichokes, asparagus, summer squash and broccoli.

You can also obtain best sources of fiber from fresh fruits, their seeds and pulp; though juicing fruits reduces their nutritional value. Try fiber-rich and low-glycemic fruits among them bananas, oranges, pears, peaches, water melon, grape fruit, green apples and berries. Lack of indigestible fiber from your diet can trigger inflammation from gut bacteria and cause chronic diseases, and not only fruits and veggies that support gut health but also probiotics like kefir, yoghurt, kim chi and sauerkraut. For instance you can choose to eat raw unmodified potato starch in that it triggers the synthesis of anti-inflammatory gut bacteria.

Going overboard with healthy fats

This applies to saturated fatty foods like coconut oil and butter alongside omega 3 fatty acids that are recommended in Ketogenic diet. Fats can strengthen your immune system and offer vitamins such as A, D and K in easily assimilated form. Though saturated fats are healthy if monitored, their excess consumption can lead to buildup of cholesterol that causes heart disease or even stroke. Research shows that high intake of saturated fats can raise LDL blood lipids that trigger cardiovascular inflammation. Regulate intake of such fats and oil to 1-2 tablespoons daily
can avoid buildup of plagues in arteries.

Other beneficial omega 3 fatty acids from foods like fish oil that is considered heart healthy ought to be monitored as excess consumption might lead to dysfunctional immune responses. A poor immunity can expose you to diseases, whereas consumption of oxidized omega-3 fats can damage your DNA. The oxidation in fish oil happens with poor quality fish oil since the omega-3 fatty acids are comprised of weak carbon double bonds. Ensure that you eat fatty fish 2-3 times a week, take few tablespoons of stabilized fish oil and eat food fortified or enriched with omega 3. Also lower intake of vegetable and oil based oils to control intake of omega 6 fats, say to a maximum of 10 grams a day.

Failure to monitor blood sugar

While it is true that while you are on a low-carb Ketogenic diet, your insulin levels and sugar tolerance should improve especially if suffering from diabetes, studies show that low-carb diets can make metabolic hormones like insulin and leptin to get out of balance. A chronic carb starvation or absence of insulin release can hinder leptin release, this hormone being the one that indicates satiety. Ever heard of carb cycling? It's advisable to eat carbs say every 5-7 days in order to maintain the cells sensitive to insulin and for the brain to be responsive to leptin hormone.

A problem can arise in case you consume a cheat meal say high carb or high-fat snack that can trigger release of excess glucose in the blood. That excess glucose can attach to protein molecules in what is referred to as glycation and lead to oxidative stress, which can eventually leads to different diseases. LDL cholesterol has a higher likelihood of being glycated and can lead to buildup of plague in the arteries or atherosclerosis. Even if you are on a low-carb diet, ensure that you regularly test your blood glucose levels. The results should help you determine your window to inflammation in your body; so try to maintain it to below 84 mg/dl.

A good way to avoid elevation of blood glucose in Ketogenic diet is to avoid high-carb cheat meals from refined foods. Instead of cheat meals or occasional high carb snacks, consider carb cycling that feature those whole unprocessed or complex carbs like fruits, squash, sweet potatoes and whole grains. It's also recommendable to have your hemoglobin A1C level determined in order to realize how your body handled glucose for the last 3 previous months. The test illustrates whether hemoglobin has been damaged by glycated glucose or not, so ensure that your results are below 5.5 percent.

Fasting while on low-carb diet

In an attempt to lose weight faster, you may want to combine a low carb diet and fasting for maximum results. While some people have experienced positive results with this combination, it may not be the best. When on a low carb diet, your sugar levels are low and your body turns to burning fat for energy. Even as you keep your sugar levels low by reducing your carbohydrate intake, it is important to avoid hypoglycemia. If you get to this point, your body will signal the adrenal glands to release cortisol and adrenaline. Cortisol, the stress hormone responsible for the "flight and fight" response will then signal the liver to convert any carbohydrates into glucose, which is then released to the blood stream. This is because your body thinks that you are in duress and you need all the glucose you can get to function. With consistently high glucose levels, your cells then crave for glucose and this can make the brain to trigger production of hormones for hunger. This will then leads to overeating, which is counterproductive.

Not getting enough essential minerals

Being on a low-carb diet and the state of ketosis can cause frequent urination, which go along with nutrients such as potassium, magnesium, and sodium. For instance electrolytes such as potassium and sodium are normally excreted along with ketones and a large amount of water as well. Lack of essential electrolytes can lead to low blood pressure, mineral imbalances and sluggishness. The symptoms of loss of electrolytes may be interpreted as low blood sugar and can cause you to give up on your low-carb diet.

The rule of the thumb during ketosis is to consume about 5000mg sodium daily, 300mg of magnesium and 100grams of potassium. A healthy diet can help you compensate for mineral requirements but in some cases, there's no need to take mineral supplements. On the other hand, supplementing with magnesium can lead to more complications for those people with kidney problems. Remember that magnesium is a co-factor in more than 300
enzymes in your body, and helps regulate a number of biochemical functions in your body. Magnesium is also required by the body to synthesize DNA and monitor heartbeat rate.

To increase the level of magnesium in the body, try using a cup of soymilk, ½ cup of boiled spinach, a medium banana, ½ cup of black beans and an ounce of cashew-nuts or almonds, roasted. And to get required potassium, ensure that you consume green veggies and also cook your meats together with broths. For sodium, you only need 2.5 to 3.5 grams of sodium so don't eat packaged or processed foods as these could be overloaded with sodium.

Not staying hydrated

A basic fact is that carbs attract water and facilitate the body to remain hydrated, and thus a low-carb diet can cause dehydration and strain the kidneys. Water also helps flush out toxins from the kidney and facilitate weight loss as toxins as usually stored as fat leading to weight gain. Many dieters on low-carb diet are afraid of water retention and thus regulate water intake in a bid to see immediate results on the scale. Though instant weight loss can impress you to stick to low-carb diet, the body quickly adjusts and instead adopts other ways of water retention. Did you know that dehydration also triggers cravings? It can also interrupt beta-oxidation process that deals with metabolism of fats as energy sources. In case you regularly take a few cups of coffee daily, ensure you also consume a few glasses say 6-8 of pure and plain water as well. And for beer lovers, it's good that you moderate your intake or avoid alcohol altogether, even whisky or red wine!

Having too many cheat days

Let's face it, it can be hard to fully forsake your sweet tooth, and thus occasionally you can choose to eat a few sugary snacks. However, eating a high carb snack hinders ketosis and slows down weight loss. Furthermore, carbs (especially simple carbs) cause cravings for more carbs as it alters your brain's hunger detention mechanism! The key is to try harder not to cheat and also avoiding those packaged low-carb foods as they are likely to be loaded with sugar alcohol. This substance is an addictive that can elevate sugar level in your metabolism due to its high glycemic index. Using such packed "healthy" products can cause hormonal imbalance and hinder effective weight loss.

You can adopt various creative ways to snack and enjoy what you eat without going overboard, if only you have prepared snacks regularly. For instance, the protein-rich nuts, hard cheese slices, or hard-boiled eggs can come in handy. Normally, we would want to have a cheat meal especially when we don't have much to eat around the house. Therefore, avoid these instances by ensuring that there is always a healthy meal. Did you know that leftovers could help simplify your life especially if served as lunch or snack? Therefore, always have some leftovers for the following day to ensure that you always have healthy foods at hand and this will avoid instances of wanting a cheat meal.

Also ensure that you eat at least 2 low-carb snacks per day especially after breakfast, after lunch and dinner, to help remain fuller. For additional snack options, try taking nuts, tuna, smoked salmon, hard-boiled eggs, leftover diced pork chops, leftover pulled chicken or taco meat. Ensure to use fats when dressing salads; and use enzyme-rich mayonnaise or sour cream combined with healthy oils for a creamy taste. Try Asian snacks among them dried anchovies and kelp chips prepared in coconut or palm oil. You can also fry your own snacks, by simply frying cheese in bacon grease or coconut oil. Also fry veggies such as peppers and onions in lard or coconut oil until crisp. Remember to add in some herbs and spices, like garlic and black pepper.

Not exercising regularly

Regardless of how a low-carb diet can facilitate detox and weight loss, you need to adopt a physically fit lifestyle as well. Research shows that altering diet only works for few dieters, and soon the body will adapt to the diet and you reach a weight loss plateau!

Exercising can help trigger synthesis of proteins and can inhibit your body from utilizing the muscle mass for fat loss. Workouts such as aerobic exercising can help the body metabolize fats for energy especially if you're already obese or living a sedentary lifestyle. Interval exercises can also help you burn fats, reduce bad cholesterol, control blood sugar and strengthen the heart and lungs. Even if you are busy most of the day, try to have at least 20 minutes of interval training per day.
Ways to exercise can involve constant movement like walking let's say amid a normal chat to a friend. Here you can do 5 minutes warm up before doing interval training; and rest for 5 minutes to allow cooling down. Alternatively, you can choose to walk at a brisk pace, where you can still manage a conversation amid breathing faster. For better results, try to move or walk at a faster pace. In case it's a weekend, try more challenging workouts like biking, swimming or other top speed activity. Ensure that once your fitness improves that you increase your speed and resistance to match your new level.

Eating excessive nuts

Nuts are good snack options and can help you avoid eating processed foods that wreck havoc on insulin production and fat metabolism. However, failure to monitor the amounts of nuts you snack on can be a problem since not all nuts are the same. For instance based on calorie levels, chestnuts, pistachios and cashew nuts are the worst in terms of their calorie content. These nuts could be full of heart-healthy fats but eating half a bag in a day can leads to giving your body excess calories than what it actually needs. You will be surprised to learn that, just 100 grams of cashew nuts has a whooping 550 calories! In case you love nuts and can't get over it, try to store them away from you; and then only carry a few with you to help track intake.

Chapter 1:
Ketogenic Diet: Triggering Weight Loss One Less Carb at a Time

The more fat you have on your body,

the longer you can survive.

If we had to rely on glucose, we'd die in a few days.

Dr. Peter Attia

Co-founder of Nutrition Science Initiative;

Ketogenic diet advocate

The ketogenic diet is a low-carbohydrate, high-fat and moderate-protein diet that aims to help people shed unwanted pounds, thus resulting to a leaner and slimmer physique. This diet focuses on reducing carbs in order to prevent the rise of blood sugar, insulin, and triglyceride levels which are the major culprits of persistent weight gain and visceral fat production.

Under the ketogenic diet, the following is a nutritional ratio that can effectively trigger fat loss and promote long-term weight management:

Fat – 150 grams per day, or 73% of total daily consumption

Protein – 90 grams per day, or 20% total daily consumption

Carbohydrates – 30 grams per day, or 7% total daily consumption

This implies that adopting a ketogenic lifestyle requires us to drastically reduce our carbohydrate intake and incorporate more healthy fats into our meals in order for the body to undergo nutritional ketosis, a process wherein the body derives energy from fat cells instead of sugar.

The Science behind Ketosis and Weight Loss

Once the body starts to consume fewer carbohydrates from food such as rice, bread or potatoes, lesser glucose is released into the bloodstream. High levels or blood sugar and insulin, the body's conventional sources of fuel, are dramatically reduced. At this stage, transitioning to a ketogenic diet may initially cause weakness and intense cravings as energy sources within the body change.

However, the absence of carbs and sugars subsequently allows nutritional ketosis to take over the energy production process within the body. The moment that stored bodily fat cells are broken into energy, the body becomes leaner, lighter and more effective at performing weight loss activities such as cardio exercises and weight training

Moreover, once the body becomes ketogenic-adapted, you will find that cravings for carbohydrates will reduce and the body will be looking forward to eating cleaner and healthier food such as vegetables, fruits, meat and oils. As a result, symptoms of lifestyle diseases such as diabetes, heart disease, chronic pain and obesity will become easier to manage or eliminate.

Based on the natural effects of ketosis, the ketogenic diet is a more effective weight loss tool than other low-carb or calorie-restrictive diets: it does not only trigger fat loss and high energy levels but it also prevents the onset of medical conditions that threaten people's health and longevity. Through proper nutrition and smarter food choices, the ketogenic diet will help the body achieve a total transformation which will significantly improve the quality of life.

Foods to Eat For Effective Ketosis

People who are unfamiliar with the ketogenic diet tend to pre-judge this healthy meal plan as difficult to maintain mainly because organic foods are seemingly hard to find and a bit more expensive than the usual items seen at the grocery store.

On the contrary, a ketogenic meal plan consists of low-carb vegetables, eggs, dairy, fruits, meats, seafood and healthy oils that can be easily found in the outer lanes of the grocery or among the colorful, healthy crates of organic
food items at your local market. Natural spices and organic sweeteners can be used to add flare to ketogenic recipes, hence making these dishes more flavorful than your usual take-outs or microwaveable dinners.

Moreover, organic ingredients are reasonably-priced in comparison with high-carb meal options such as rice dinners, boxed pizza or fast food. Apart from saving you money, a keto lifestyle also promotes creativity in the kitchen by encouraging you to combine cheap but healthy ingredients in order to create a weight-friendly daily meal plan.

While organic food are at the top of the list, the ketogenic diet discourages the high consumption of natural carbs such as rice, high-carb vegetables, bread, grains, fruits and legumes as these tend to spike-up blood sugar levels. It is important to keep the carbohydrate ratio low so that you do not fall off the ketogenic wagon and gain even more weight.

The succeeding chapter contains a complete one-week meal plan that will serve as your initial guide in ketogenic meal preparation. Hopefully this will help you in your journey towards healthier living and long-term weight loss.

Chapter 2:
Comprehensive 7-Day Ketogenic Meal Plan for Beginners

Creating a weekly ketogenic meal plan may take a bit more time than the usual, but once you master the carbohydrate-fat-protein ratio then you will find that transitioning to a keto lifestyle is as simple as adopting a portion-controlled, organic way eating.

Here is a comprehensive 7-day ketogenic meal plan that will give you an idea on how to create a balanced set of nutritious dishes throughout the day.

Day 1

Breakfast – Parmesan, Ham and Basil Omelet

Lunch – Keto-Friendly Fried Chicken

Snack – Spicy Baked Zucchini Chips

Dinner – Coconut Fish Fingers with Garlic Mayo Dip

Dessert – Frozen Watermelon Creamsicles

Day 2

Breakfast – Spicy and Savory Breakfast Patties

Lunch – Fiery Egg Drop Soup

Snack – Baked Coconut Crisps

Dinner – Wheat-Free Pork and Veggie Sandwich

Dessert – Luscious Coconut Brownies

Day 3

Breakfast – High-Fiber Keto Oatmeal

Lunch – Low-Carb Tuna Avocado Meatballs

Snack – Garlicky Pork Chips

Dinner – Oven-Baked Rib-eye Steak

Dessert – Coconut Pudding with Fresh Berries

Day 4

Breakfast – Energizer Green Smoothie

Lunch – Spiced Pork Chops with Stir-Fried Veggies

Snack – Crispy Brussels Sprouts with Hot Mayo Sauce

Dinner – Low-Carb Vegetarian Pan Pizza

Dessert – Watermelon & Cucumber Sorbet

Day 5

Breakfast – Fully Loaded Breakfast Frittata

Lunch – Low-Carb Bacon Meatball Skewers

Snack – Light and Healthy Spinach Crackers

Dinner – Grilled Tilapia Fillet with Arugula Salad

Dessert – Almond Coconut Fat Bombs

Day 6

Breakfast – Crunchy Sunflower Seed Cereal

Lunch – Low-Carb Zucchini Carbonara

Snack – Cheesy Baked Sugar Snap Peas

Dinner – Quick and Easy Grilled Chicken Teriyaki

Dessert – Heavenly Chocolate Bacon Strips

Day 7

Breakfast – Sunny Tangerine Smoothie

Lunch – Summer Tomato, Cucumber and Shrimp Salad

Snack – Extra Spicy Devilled Eggs

Dinner – Slow-Braised Oxtail Stew

Dessert – Chocolate Peppermint Bark

The complete recipes of the dishes listed on this 7-day meal plan are found on the succeeding chapters. In addition, there are 35 more ketogenic recipes included in this book in order to give you more options and creativity for your meals.

Chapter 3:
Breakfast Recipes

Make yourself a low-carb breakfast such as scrambled eggs, lean meat burgers or fruit smoothies: this will provide you with intense energy throughout the day and supply your body with the right nutrients needed for that morning workout.

1. <u>Parmesan, Ham and Basil Omelet</u>

Ingredients:

4 large eggs

1½ tablespoons freshly-chopped basil leaves

¾ cup grated parmesan cheese

2 thin slices of cooked ham, minced

1 small avocado, pitted and sliced

2 tablespoons coconut oil

Pinch of sea salt

Directions:

Whisk together the eggs and parmesan cheese. Add in the basil, ham and sea salt. Mix well.

Heat the coconut oil in a pan over medium-high flame. Once the oil is hot, pour in the egg mixture and cook for 30 seconds. To prevent the egg from burning, use a spatula to push the sides of the egg towards the center.

Flip the omelet and cook the other side for 1 minute. Once the omelet is cooked, remove it from the heat and transfer it to a serving plate.

Top the omelet with avocado slices and serve.

This recipe yields 2 servings.

2. <u>Sunny Tangerine Smoothie</u>

Ingredients:

3 cups full-fat coconut milk

4 tablespoons shredded coconut

5 tangerines, peeled and deseeded

2 teaspoons tangerine zest

½cup fresh lime juice

½teaspoon vanilla

3 cups ice cubes

Directions:

Pour the coconut milk and lime juice in a blender and pulse. Add in the shredded coconut, tangerines, zest, vanilla and ice cubes and blend the smoothie for 10-15 seconds.

Pour the smoothie into glasses and serve immediately.

This recipe yields 4 servings.

3. **Energizer Green Smoothie**

Ingredients:
1 avocado, peeled, pitted and sliced

3 cups spinach leaves

1½ tablespoons roasted flaxseed

1½ cups almond milk

1 cup coconut milk

4 drops liquid stevia

3 ice cubes

Directions:

Place the avocado, spinach, flaxseed, almond milk, coconut milk, stevia and ice cubes in a blender and process until the desired consistency is met.

Pour the smoothie into glasses and serve immediately.

This recipe yields 2 servings.

4. **Microwaveable Bacon and Egg Biscuit**

Ingredients:

2 large eggs

4 tablespoon flaxseed meal

2 tablespoons coconut flour

2 teaspoons unsalted butter

1 teaspoon baking powder

Pinch of sea salt

3 bacon strips, cooked until golden brown

2 sunny-side up cooked eggs

Directions:

In a mixing bowl, blend together the flour, flaxseed, salt and baking powder. Add in the butter and slowly mix it into the flour mixture with a fork. The flour mixture should have a crumbly appearance.

Beat 2 large eggs in a separate bowl then slowly pour into the flour mixture. With a wooden spoon, mix the ingredients together until a smooth batter forms.

Divide the batter by pouring it into 2 greased 4-inch ramekins. Place the ramekins in a microwave and cook it on high for 1 minute. Once the biscuits are done, let it cool then remove it from the ramekins.

Slice each biscuit vertically in the middle. Place equal amounts of bacon and egg in between each biscuit then serve immediately.

This recipe yields 2 servings.

5. Savory Green Waffles

Ingredients:

1 bunch spinach, washed, drained and chopped

4 eggs

3 bacon strips, cooked and chopped

1 tablespoon full-fat coconut milk

Pinch of salt and black pepper
Directions:

Place the coconut milk and eggs in a bowl then whisk them together. Gradually fold in the chopped spinach and mix well. Season the egg mixture with salt and pepper.

Grease the waffle iron with cooking spray and turn on the heat. Pour the egg mixture into the heated pan and sprinkle chopped bacon on top. Close the waffle iron and let the dish cook for 3 minutes. Once the waffle is cooked, use a fork to remove it from the pan and transfer it to a serving plate.

This recipe yields 2 servings.

6. **Early Riser's Muffin Sandwich**

Ingredients:

4 large eggs

200 grams breakfast sausage

½ cup chicken stock

4 tablespoons melted unsalted butter

Pinch of sea salt and black pepper

Hot sauce

Directions:

To make the muffin loaves, pour 2 tablespoons of butter on a frying pan over medium flame. Once the butter begins to heat up, place 4 round biscuit cutters on the pan. Place an egg into each biscuit cutter then prick the yolks with a fork. Sprinkle each egg with salt and pepper.

Slowly pour the chicken stock into the pan, making sure that the liquid stays outside the biscuit cutters. Cover the pan, adjust the flame to low and cook the eggs for 3-4 minutes. Once the eggs are cooked, slowly remove them from the pan and let it cool.

To make the sausage patty, pour the remaining butter onto the pan and heat it up over medium flame. Create 2 thick and round patties with the breakfast sausage then place them on the pan. Cook each side for 3 minutes.

To assemble the sandwich, place 2 eggs on a plate. Place a sausage patty over each egg, squeeze some hot sauce over it then cover each patty with the remaining eggs.

This recipe yields 2 servings.

7. **Crunchy Sunflower Seed Cereal**

Ingredients:

1 ½ cups raw sunflower seeds

1 ½ tablespoons ground cinnamon

2 cups coconut shreds

1 teaspoon coconut oil

½teaspoon sea salt

2 medium eggs

½cup organic honey

2 cups full-fat coconut milk, chilled

Directions:

Prepare a parchment-lined baking sheet and preheat the oven to 350 ° F.

Grind the sunflower seeds and coconut shreds in a food processor. Once both ingredients are fully chopped, add in the eggs, honey, salt, cinnamon and coconut oil. Process the mixture for 1-2 minutes.

Using a spatula, place the mixture into the baking sheet and press downwards and sideways for an even thickness. Place the cereal in the oven and bake for 15 minutes.

Once the cereal is ready, remove it from the oven and let it cool for 20 minutes. Use a wooden spoon to lightly tap and break the cereal into small bits.

Place the cereal into individual bowls and pour the chilled coconut milk on top of it. Serve immediately.

This recipe makes 2 servings.

8. Keto-Friendly Pancakes and Bacon Strips

Ingredients:

10 bacon slices, cooked

1 cup almond flour

½cup coconut flour

5 large eggs

½ teaspoon baking soda ¼ cup coconut milk

¼ cup water

12 drops liquid stevia ¼ cup Erythritol

¼ cup egg white protein

½ cup melted unsalted butter Directions:

Whisk together the eggs, coconut milk, water and liquid stevia. Set this aside.

In another bowl, mix together the almond flour, coconut flour, baking soda, Erythritol and egg white protein.

Slowly pour the egg mixture into the dry ingredients. Mix the pancake batter thoroughly.

Heat the butter in a pan over medium flame. Using a wooden spoon, pour a strip of batter into the pan, making sure its shape mimics the shape of the bacon strip. Place a strip of bacon in the middle of the pancake and wait for the sides to bubble. Flip the pancake and continue cooking for a minute or two. Follow the same process for the remaining batter until you have 10 bacon pancakes. Serve warm.

This recipe yields 5 servings.

9. <u>Spicy and Savory Breakfast Patties</u>

Ingredients:

900 grams ground chicken meat

1 large egg, beaten

1 teaspoon garlic powder

2 teaspoon sea salt

1 teaspoon onion powder

½ teaspoon fresh thyme ¼ teaspoon chili flakes

1 teaspoon ground black pepper

1 teaspoon chopped parsley ¼ teaspoon nutmeg

¼ teaspoon paprika

2 teaspoons chopped dried sage

3 tablespoons olive oil

Directions:

Place the ground chicken and egg in a bowl and mix well. Gradually blend in the garlic powder, salt, onion powder, thyme, sage, nutmeg, paprika and chili flakes into the chicken mixture. Form the spiced mixture into 16 round patties then set aside.

Heat the olive oil in a pan over medium flame. Place the patties on the hot oil and cook for 3-5 minutes. Flip each patty over and cook the remaining side for 3 minutes. Place the breakfast patties on a plate and serve while hot.

This recipe yields 8 servings.

10. <u>Fruit and Greens Breakfast Bowl</u>

Ingredients:

2 cups kale leaves, stems discarded

2 scoops protein powder

4 tablespoons coconut cream

1 cup almond milk

2 tablespoons melted coconut oil

4 ice cubes

1 tablespoon shredded coconut

2 tablespoons ground almonds

2 teaspoons chia seeds

Slices of banana

Directions:

Place the kale leaves, whey protein, coconut cream, almond milk, coconut oil and ice cubes in a blender.
Process for 20 seconds then pour the contents in a bowl.

Sprinkle the ground almonds, shredded coconut and chia seeds on top of the cereal. Top with banana slices and serve.

This recipe yields 2 servings.

11. Herbed Bacon and Egg Cups

Ingredients:

½tablespoon chopped fresh chives

½tablespoon chopped fresh parsley

12 bacon strips

8 eggs

½cup cottage cheese

½cup shredded cheddar cheese

2 jalapeno peppers, deseeded and minced

½ teaspoon garlic powder

Pinch of salt and ground black pepper
Olive oil

Directions:

Lightly grease 12 muffin cups with olive oil and set aside. Preheat the oven to 350 ° F.

Place the bacon in a pan over medium flame and cook until light golden brown but not crispy. Cool the bacon for 2 minutes, then place a strip inside each muffin cup, circling the sides of the vessel. Set aside.

Whisk together the eggs, chives, parsley, cheeses, jalapeno peppers, garlic powder, salt and pepper in a mixing bowl. Pour the egg mixture into each bacon-lined cup, making sure that some space is left on the top so as to prevent the egg from overflowing.

Bake the egg cups for 25 minutes. Serve immediately.

This recipe yields 12 servings.

12.   High-Fiber Keto Oatmeal

Ingredients:

4 cups coconut milk

¾ cup flaxseeds

1 cup ground almonds

½cup finely-chopped cauliflower

½cup cottage cheese

¼ cup heavy cream

3 tablespoons unsalted butter, melted

1 teaspoon cinnamon powder

¼ teaspoon allspice ½ teaspoon vanilla ½ teaspoon nutmeg

10 drops liquid stevia

3 tablespoons Erythritol Directions:

Pour the coconut milk inside a saucepan and mix in the cauliflower. Heat the mixture over medium-high flame.

Once the mixture starts to boil, season it with cinnamon, allspice, vanilla and nutmeg. Mix well. Gradually add in the stevia, Erythritol and flaxseeds and mix until the oatmeal starts to thicken.

Pour the melted butter, cottage cheese and heavy cream into the oatmeal mixture and continue cooking for 5 minutes. Turn off the heat then spoon the oatmeal into individual bowls. Sprinkle chopped almonds on top of each bowl of oatmeal. Serve while hot.

This recipe yields 6 servings.

13.   Bacon and Eggs in a Basket

Ingredients:

7 medium eggs

7 bacon slices, chopped

1 cup finely-chopped tomatoes

2 cups grated sharp cheddar cheese

3 tablespoons olive oil

½ teaspoon salt

1 teaspoon paprika

½ teaspoon cayenne pepper Directions:

Preheat the oven to 400 ° F and line a baking sheet with parchment paper. Prepare an upside down muffin tin that will mold the cheese baskets.

To make the baskets, place 7 equal mounds of cheddar cheese on the baking sheet and sprinkle it with cayenne pepper and paprika. Bake the cheese mounds in the oven for 10 minutes.

Remove the cheese from the oven and slowly place them on top of the upside-down muffin pan, letting the sides fall slightly but not detach from the base. Let it cool and harden at room temperature.

While the cheese baskets are setting, heat the olive oil in a pan over medium-high flame. Fry each egg in a sunny-side up manner then set aside. Sprinkle some salt over each egg.

Once the eggs are done, cook the chopped bacon in the same pan until it becomes golden brown.

To assemble the dish, place 1 cheese basket on a plate. Place an egg over the basket followed by half a teaspoon of bacon. Top each basket with some chopped tomatoes and serve immediately.

This recipe yields 7 servings.

14. **Fully-Loaded Breakfast Frittata**

Ingredients:

12 eggs

2 cups sharp cheddar cheese, grated

6 cups kale leaves, washed and drained

1 small onion, chopped

1 green bell pepper, deseeded and chopped

4 tablespoons coconut milk

4 tablespoons heavy cream

200 grams breakfast sausage

200 grams chorizo, casing discarded

1 teaspoon garlic powder

1 tablespoon olive oil

Pinch of sea salt

Directions:

Place the kale leaves, onions, bell peppers and olive oil in a pan and cook the vegetables on medium-high flame for 5 minutes. Remove the veggies from the heat and transfer it to a large mixing bowl.

In the same pan, cook together the sausage and chorizo until the meat becomes golden brown. Once the meat is cooked, transfer it into the bowl of cooked vegetables. Add in the cheddar cheese and mix the ingredients together. Set aside.

Whisk together the eggs, coconut milk and heavy cream. Season it with garlic powder and salt. Pour the egg mixture into the bowl of vegetables, cheese and meat. Blend the ingredients well.

Pour the frittata mixture into a lightly greased skillet and place it in the oven. Bake the frittata for 45 minutes inside a 350 ° F oven.

Let the frittata cool for 10 minutes then slice into squares. Serve warm.

This recipe yields 20 servings.

Chapter 4:
Lunch Recipes

B reak that mid-day hunger by eating a light, ketogenic lunch. Whether you have a veggie salad, soup or a plate of lean pork chops, a low-carb lunch will help keep the stomach full and maintain energy for mid-day activities such as lunch meetings or household chores.

1.   **Spiced Pork Chops with Stir-Fried Veggies**

Ingredients:

3 large pork chops

2 teaspoons cumin

1 teaspoon coriander

1 teaspoon garlic powder

¼ cup flaxseed

Pinch of salt and ground black pepper

1 yellow bell pepper, deseeded and chopped

2 celery stalks, chopped

1 white onion, chopped

1 tablespoon butter

3 tablespoons olive oil

Directions:

In a bowl, mix together the cumin, coriander, flaxseed and garlic powder. Dip each pork chop into the spice mixture, making sure that all sides are evenly coated. Set aside.

Heat the olive oil in a pan over medium-high flame. Add the pork chops to the hot oil and cook for 3-5 minutes. Flip the pork chops over and cook the other side for 3 minutes. Remove the meat from the heat and let it cool for 5 minutes.

In another pan, heat the butter over medium flame. Add in the celery, bell peppers and onions and stir-fry the vegetables for 3 minutes. Turn off the heat.

Place the stir-fried vegetables on a plate. Arrange the pork chops on top of the vegetables. Serve immediately.

This recipe yields 3 servings.

2. Keto-Friendly Egg Salad

Ingredients:

3 pre-boiled eggs, cooled and peeled

3 lettuce leaves (Romaine or Iceberg)

1 teaspoon Dijon mustard

½teaspoon fresh lemon juice

1 ½ tablespoon mayonnaise

1 teaspoon olive oil

½teaspoon paprika

Pinch of salt and ground black pepper

Directions:

Place the eggs in a food processor and pulse until the eggs are roughly chopped. Gradually mix in the mayonnaise, mustard and lemon juice then blend for 10 seconds. Open the food processor then season the egg mixture with paprika, salt and pepper. Blend the salad for 5-10 seconds, depending on the preferred creaminess of the mixture.

Arrange the lettuce leaves on a serving plate. Spoon the egg salad onto the bed of lettuce then drizzle olive oil on top before serving.

This recipe yields 2 servings.

3. Fiery Egg Drop Soup

Ingredients:

4 eggs

3 cups homemade chicken broth

1 cup coconut milk

1 tablespoon butter

½ chicken bouillon

1 ½ teaspoons red chili flakes

Directions:

In a large saucepan over medium-high flame, boil together the chicken broth, bouillon and butter. Stir occasionally. Lower the flame once the stock starts to bubble.

One by one, crack the eggs into the steaming stock. Pour in the coconut milk then season it with red chili flakes. Stir the soup for 2 minutes then turn off the flame. Continue stirring for another 2 minutes or until the soup starts to thicken. Pour into bowls and serve while hot.

This recipe yields 4 servings.

4. Chunky Avocado and Tomato Salad

Ingredients:

2 large avocadoes, peeled and pitted

500 grams tomatoes

4 cups chopped lettuce

10 bacon slices, fried and chopped

¾ cup mayonnaise

Pinch of salt and black pepper

Directions:

Slice the avocadoes and tomatoes into ½ inch chunks and place them in a salad bowl. Mix in the lettuce and mayonnaise then toss the ingredients together. Season the salad with salt and pepper. Sprinkle the chopped bacon on top before serving.

This recipe yields 4 servings.

5. Summer Tomato, Cucumber and Shrimp Salad

Ingredients:

1 heirloom tomato, diced

450 grams cooked shrimp, diced

1 medium cucumber, peeled and diced
 1 tablespoon bottled capers

2 tablespoons mayonnaise

2 teaspoons Dijon mustard

½ cup lemon juice

Pinch of sea salt and black pepper

½teaspoon fresh dill

2 cups mixed greens Directions:

Arrange the mixed greens in a salad bowl and set aside.

In a separate bowl, toss together the tomatoes, cucumbers, shrimp, capers, mustard, mayonnaise and lemon juice. Season the tossed salad with salt and pepper.

Pour the salad into the bowl of mixed greens and sprinkle fresh dill on top. Chill the salad in the refrigerator for an hour then serve.

This recipe yields 3 servings.

6. Keto-Friendly Fried Chicken

Ingredients:

2 chicken breasts, sliced and opened up

2 large eggs, beaten

¾cup shredded parmesan cheese

1 cup ground pork rinds

2 tablespoons coconut oil

Pinch of salt and ground black pepper Directions:

Mix together the parmesan, pork rinds, salt and pepper in a bowl.

In a separate bowl, place the beaten eggs. Heat the coconut oil in a pan over medium-high flame.

Dip each chicken breast into the egg mixture then place it into the pork rind bowl to coat it. After that, dip the chicken into the egg mixture again and roll it into the rind mixture.

Place the coated chicken into the pan of hot oil and cook each side for 6-8 minutes. You may lower the heat once you have flipped the chicken over.

This recipe yields 2 servings.

7. Low-Carb Tuna Avocado Meatballs

Ingredients:

280 grams canned tuna fish, drained

1 medium avocado, peeled, pitted and diced

1 cup chopped celery

¼cup cottage cheese

¼cup mayonnaise

¼teaspoon onion powder

¼teaspoon paprika
 1/3 cup almond flour

1 cup olive oil

Pinch of salt and ground black pepper

Directions:

Transfer the tuna to a mixing bowl and season it with salt, onion powder, paprika and pepper. Mix well.

Add in the avocado, celery, cheese and mayonnaise. Slightly mash the ingredients together. Form 12 meatballs from the tuna avocado mixture then roll it in the almond flour. Set aside.

Heat the olive oil in a pan over medium-high flame. Once the oil is hot, fry the meatballs until the sides are golden brown. Let it cool for 5 minutes then serve.

This recipe yields 12 meatballs

8. <u>Hot and Spicy Pork Taco Wraps</u>

Ingredients:

10 iceberg or Boston lettuce leaves, washed and drained

400 grams lean ground pork

1 cup tomato salsa

½ teaspoon garlic powder ¼ teaspoon cumin

½teaspoon onion powder

¼teaspoon ground black pepper

1 tablespoon olive oil

Slices of avocado, bell peppers and red onions Directions:

Place the ground pork, garlic powder, cumin, onion powder and black pepper in a bowl. Using your hands, knead the spices into the meat.

Heat the olive oil in a skillet over medium flame. Place the spiced ground pork on the skillet and cook it until the meat becomes brown.

Once the meat is cooked, turn off the flame and drain the excess oil from the cooked pork. Pour the salsa over the pork and mix well.

To assemble the taco wraps, place a lettuce leaf on a plate, spoon the pork mixture on top of it then place some chopped avocadoes, peppers and onions. Fold or roll the lettuce leaf to secure the pork inside it. Serve immediately.

This recipe yields 2 servings.

9. <u>Low-Carb Bacon Meatball Skewers</u>

Ingredients:

5 bacon slices

450 grams ground pork

½teaspoon salt

½teaspoon ground black pepper

½teaspoon onion powder

½teaspoon garlic powder
½ teaspoon turmeric powder

½cup olive oil

Chunks of tomato, cucumber and pineapple

Directions:

Place the bacon and ground pork in a food processor and blend well. Season the meatball mixture with salt, pepper, onion powder, garlic powder and turmeric powder.

Form the mixture into 20 meatballs and place it on a parchment-lined baking sheet. Bake the meatballs in a 170 ° F oven for 12 minutes. Let the meatballs cool on a wire rack for 10 minutes.

To serve, place a chunk of tomato, cucumber, pineapple and meatball through a small skewer. Place the skewers on a serving plate and drizzle with olive oil.

This recipe yields 10 servings.

10. __Zesty Chili Crab Cakes__

Ingredients:

3 cups fresh crab meat

2 large eggs

2 tablespoon coconut flour

4 tablespoons minced green chilies

1 tablespoon minced garlic

1 teaspoon Dijon mustard

½ teaspoon mayonnaise

Pinch of sea salt and black pepper

3 tablespoons olive oil

Directions:

In a large bowl, mix together the crab meat, eggs, chilies, garlic, mustard and mayonnaise. Season the mixture with salt and pepper then gradually add the coconut flour to thicken its consistency. Mix well.

Form the mixture into 10 round patties and set aside.

Heat the olive oil in a large pan over medium-high flame. Place the crab cakes on the pan and cook each side for 3 minutes or until golden brown.

This recipe yields 10 servings.

11. <u>Crunchy Greens and Pine Nuts Salad</u>

Ingredients:

Directions:

1 cup arugula

1 cup spinach

3 iceberg lettuce leaves, torn

3 tablespoons toasted pine nuts

3 bacon slices, cooked

1 cup shredded parmesan cheese

2 tablespoons lemon juice
2 tablespoons olive oil

Pinch of salt and ground black pepper

Directions:

Wash and pat dry the arugula, spinach and lettuce leaves. Place them in a salad bowl.

Chop the bacon into small pieces then add these on top of the greens. Sprinkle the pine nuts and parmesan cheese on top of the salad. Set aside.

In a small bowl, whisk together the olive oil, lemon juice, salt and pepper. Pour the dressing into the salad bowl and toss the ingredients together. Place the salad in the refrigerator for 1 hour.

This recipe yields 3 servings.

12. <u>Roasted Cauliflower and Pepper Chowder</u>

Ingredients:

1 small head of cauliflower, cut into small florets

2 green bell peppers, halved and deseeded

3 green onions, minced

2 tablespoons olive oil

4 tablespoons butter

½teaspoon red pepper flakes

½cup coconut cream

3 cups homemade chicken broth

1 teaspoon garlic powder

1 teaspoon paprika

1 teaspoon chopped fresh thyme

Pinch of salt and ground black pepper

Directions:

Preheat the oven to 400 ° F and line 2 baking sheets with parchment paper.

Arrange the pepper halves on a baking sheet. Meanwhile, place the cauliflower florets on the other baking sheet then drizzle olive oil on top. Place both baking sheets in the oven to roast the vegetables.

After 10 minutes, remove the baking sheet with the peppers from the oven. Place the peppers in a zip lock bag and leave the vegetables to sweat for 10 minutes. Take out the peppers and slowly peel off the skin. Slice the peppers into strips and set aside.

After 30 minutes, take out the roasted cauliflower florets from the oven and set aside.

Heat the butter in a large saucepan over medium-high flame. Once the butter starts to heat up, add in the green onions, thyme, red pepper flakes, garlic powder, paprika, salt and pepper. Mix well.

Once the spices are cooked, pour in the coconut cream and chicken broth. Stir and let the mixture simmer. Add in the cauliflower and peppers and simmer for 10 minutes before turning off the heat.

Pour the chowder into a blender and pulse a few times. If you want the chowder to come out smoother, blend the mixture for 15 seconds. Pour into bowls and serve immediately.

This recipe yields 5 servings.

13. <u>Low-Carb Zucchini Carbonara</u>

Ingredients:
3 medium zucchinis, peeled

1 cup chopped bacon

3 tablespoons freshly-chopped basil leaves

½cup grated parmesan cheese

1 egg

2 egg yolks, beaten

2 tablespoons heavy cream

Pinch of salt and ground black pepper Directions:

Place the zucchinis through a spiralizer to form long, spaghetti-like noodles. Transfer the noodles to a bowl and set aside.

Fry the chopped bacon in a pan over medium-high flame until golden brown. Remove the bacon but save the bacon fat for later.

Whisk together the egg and egg yolks and season it with salt and pepper. Blend in the parmesan cheese and heavy cream then set aside.

Place the zucchini noodles in the pan of bacon fat and cook over medium-high flame for 5 minutes. Add the egg mixture then cook for 2-3 minutes with constant stirring. Turn off the heat and transfer the pasta to a serving plate.

Top the dish with bacon bits and serve immediately.

This recipe yields 3 servings.

14. <u>Pan-Fried Salmon with Zesty Balsamic Sauce</u>

Ingredients:

2 150-gram salmon fillets

2 tablespoons white wine

1 tablespoon organic ketchup

1 tablespoon fish sauce

2 teaspoons olive oil

2 tablespoons coconut aminos

1 tablespoon balsamic vinegar

2 teaspoons chopped garlic

1 teaspoon chopped ginger

2 teaspoons organic honey

Directions:

Mix together coconut aminos, honey, fish sauce, balsamic vinegar, garlic and ginger in a bowl. Place the salmon fillets in the balsamic mixture and marinate for 15 minutes.

After 15 minutes, drain the liquid from the salmon fillets and set aside.

Heat the olive oil in a pan over medium-high flame. Once the oil is hot, place the salmon fillets on the pan, skin side down. Fry for 3 minutes, then slowly flip the fillets and cook for another 3 minutes. Pour the balsamic marinade into the pan and let it boil with the fish.

Take out the fried fish from the pan and set aside. Pour the ketchup and white wine into the boiling marinade and cook for 5 minutes or until the sauce has reduced. Turn off the heat and cool for 5 minutes.

Place the salmon fillets on a plate and drizzle the sauce over it. Serve immediately.

This recipe yields 2 servings.

Chapter 5:
Dinner Recipes

Dinners are important in a ketogenic lifestyle: healthy dishes that are high in healthy fats will help keep you full throughout the night, thus preventing you from giving into cravings for high-carb midnight snacks.

1. Quick and Easy Grilled Chicken Teriyaki

Ingredients:

2 chicken breasts, skin removed

1 tablespoon olive oil

½ cup water

2 tablespoons organic honey

1 cup coconut aminos

1 teaspoon freshly-grated ginger

1 teaspoon garlic powder

Pinch of salt

Directions:

Pat the chicken breasts dry with a kitchen towel. Drizzle olive oil all over the chicken then place them on a grill pan. Cook each side of the chicken for 8-10 minutes over medium-high flame then set aside.

Whisk together water, honey, coconut aminos, ginger, garlic powder and salt in a saucepan and place the teriyaki mixture over medium flame. Boil the sauce for 7-10 minutes while constantly stirring it. Turn off the flame once the sauce has reduced.

Transfer the chicken breasts into the saucepan. Make sure to coat all side of the chicken with the teriyaki sauce. Arrange the chicken on a serving plate and serve with your favorite greens.

This recipe yields 2 servings.

2. Slow-Braised Oxtail Stew

Ingredients:

900 grams oxtail, sliced

2 cups homemade chicken broth

3 tablespoons tomato paste

3 garlic cloves, crushed

2 tablespoons coconut aminos

½ cup butter

1 teaspoon onion powder

1 teaspoon turmeric powder

Pinch of salt and ground black pepper

Directions:

Arrange the sliced oxtail in a crock pot and season it with onion powder, turmeric powder, salt, pepper and crushed garlic. Pour in the chicken broth, coconut aminos and tomato paste.

Cover the crock pot and set the temperature to low. Cook the meat for 7 hours.

Place the cooked oxtails on a serving bowl. Use an immersion blender to puree the braising liquid inside the
 pot. Pour the sauce over the oxtail slices and serve while hot.

This recipe makes 4 servings.

3. **Wheat-Free Pork and Veggie Sandwich**

Ingredients:

900 grams lean ground pork

½ cup tomato sauce

1 large white onion, minced

2 eggs

Slices of tomato and cucumber

1½ tablespoons melted butter

½teaspoon paprika

½ teaspoon chili powder Pinch of salt and black pepper Directions:

Place the chopped onions in a pan over medium-high heat then pour in the melted butter. Cook the onions for 3 minutes then let it cool.

In a large bowl, mix together the pork, tomato sauce, eggs and cooked onions. Season it with salt, pepper, chili powder and paprika then mix thoroughly. Divide the pork mixture into 6 patties and place them on a parchment-lined baking sheet. Bake the patties in a 350 ° F oven for 45 minutes.

Once the patties are cooked, remove it from the oven and allow them to cool. Slice each patty horizontally in the middle to make 2 loaves. Place a patty slice on a plate, top with cucumbers and tomatoes then cover it with the other patty. Serve immediately.

This recipe yields 6 servings.

4. Grilled Tilapia Fillet with Arugula Salad

Ingredients:

3 Tilapia fillets

2 tablespoons lime zest

1 teaspoon sea salt

1 tablespoon lemon pepper seasoning

1 teaspoon garlic powder

1 tablespoon melted coconut oil

2 cups arugula, washed and drained

1 tablespoon lemon juice

1 tablespoon olive oil

1 teaspoon honey

Directions:

To make the arugula salad, mix together the arugula leaves, lemon juice, olive oil and honey until the leaves are well-coated. Set this aside.

In another bowl, combine the lime zest, sea salt, lemon pepper seasoning and garlic powder. Place the tilapia fillets into the spice mixture and coat evenly.
 Grease the grill pan with the coconut oil and place it over medium-high flame. Place the tilapia on the grill pan and cook each side for 3-5 minutes.

Once the fillets are cooked, arrange them on a serving plate. Serve the tilapia with the prepared arugula salad.

This recipe yields 3 servings.

5. Slow Cooker Roast Beef with Honey Citrus Sauce

Ingredients:

900 grams beef chuck roast

2 tablespoons fresh lime juice

2 tablespoons fresh orange juice

1 tablespoon honey

½ cup olive oil

3 garlic cloves, minced

½cup chopped cilantro

1 large shallot, minced

1 teaspoon chili powder

2 teaspoons oregano powder

2 teaspoons sea salt ¼ teaspoon cumin ¼ teaspoon coriander ¼ cup water Directions:

Place the beef chuck inside the slow cooker. Let it stand for 20-30 minutes.

In a food processor, mix together the lime juice, orange juice, honey, olive oil, cilantro, shallot, chili powder, oregano, salt, cumin and coriander. Pour the mixture into the pot, making sure to coat the beef evenly. Pour in the water then cover the pot.

Set the temperature to high and cook the beef for 4 hours, turning the meat every hour. After 4 hours, turn off the slow cooker and tilt the cover of the pot to let the heat dissipate. Leave it for 20 minutes.

Remove the beef from the pot and place it on a serving plate. Slice the meat according to preferred thickness and pour the citrus sauce over it. Serve immediately.

This recipe yields 4-5 servings.

6. Coconut Fish Fingers with Garlic Mayo Dip

Ingredients:

450 grams cream dory, sliced into strips

¾cup shredded coconut

2 medium eggs, beaten

4 tablespoons olive oil

 Pinch of salt and black pepper For the Dip:

1 teaspoon garlic powder
3 tablespoons mayonnaise

½ teaspoon honey Directions:

Wash the fish strips and drain completely. Place the eggs in a bowl and put the shredded coconut on a separate plate.

Heat the olive oil in a pan over medium high flame.

Dip the fish finger into the egg mixture then roll it on the grated coconut. Repeat this procedure again to ensure that the fish is evenly coated.

Place the fish finger into the pan and cook until the sides have turned golden brown. Lay the fish finger on a wire rack to cool. Arrange the fish fingers on a serving plate and serve immediately.

For the dip, mix together the mayonnaise, garlic powder and honey. Pour the mixture in a sauce bowl and serve.

This recipe yields 4 servings.

7. <u>Turkey and Vegetable Pot Pie</u>

Ingredients:

1 cup leftover turkey meat, diced

1 egg, beaten

1 cup diced celery

1 cup diced zucchini

1 cup homemade chicken broth

Pinch of salt and ground black pepper

For the Crust:

2 large eggs

½ cup coconut oil 1½ cups almond flour

½ cup coconut flour Pinch of sea salt Directions:

To make the crust, combine the almond and coconut flours in a bowl then season it with salt. Add in coconut oil and egg. Knead through the mixture until a soft dough forms.

Separate the dough mixture into 2 balls. Place each dough ball in between 2 sheets of wax paper then use a rolling pin to flatten them. Place one flattened dough in a lightly-greased pie pan and spread the dough until the sides of the pan are covered. Bake this in a 325 ° F oven for 6-8 minutes.

While the pie crust is baking, place the turkey, egg, celery, zucchini and chicken broth in a saucepan and simmer over medium flame for 8 minutes. Season it with salt and pepper. Once the liquids have reduced, turn off the heat and set aside.

Once the pie crust is ready, remove it from the oven and let it cool for 3-5 minutes. Pour the turkey mixture into the pie crust. Slowly put the remaining flattened dough on top of the pie. Make sure to seal the sides of the pie but do make small vents on top by poking it with a fork or knife.

Place the pie in the oven and bake for 45-50 minutes. Slice into equal portions and serve.

This recipe yields 8 servings.

8. <u>Carb-Friendly Chili Bowl</u>

Ingredients:

900 grams ground beef

7 cups spinach leaves

1 green bell pepper, deseeded and chopped

1 red bell pepper, deseeded and chopped

1 medium onion, chopped

1 cup tomato sauce

1 tablespoon chili powder

1 tablespoon cumin

2 teaspoons cayenne pepper

1 teaspoon garlic powder

½teaspoon curry powder

1 tablespoon olive oil

2 tablespoons cottage cheese

Pinch of salt and ground black pepper Directions:

Place the ground beef in a pot and start cooking it over high flame. Stir every few minutes to prevent it from burning.

While the beef starts to cook, heat the olive oil in a large pan over medium flame. Add in the onions and bell peppers and sauté for 10 minutes. Add in the spinach leaves and cook for 10 more minutes. Season with salt and pepper and set aside.

Season the beef with chili powder, cumin, cayenne pepper, garlic powder and curry powder. Lower the flame to medium and continue cooking for 20-25 minutes.

Once the beef is cooked, add the cooked vegetables and tomato sauce into the pot and mix well. Simmer for 10 minutes then turn off the heat. Sprinkle some cottage cheese on top and serve while hot.

This recipe yields 8 servings.

9. <u>Barbecued Short Ribs with Asian Spices</u>

Ingredients:

6 short rib flanks

2 tablespoons fish sauce

2 tablespoons coconut aminos

1 tablespoon oyster sauce

2 tablespoons rice vinegar

½teaspoon red pepper flakes

1 teaspoon minced ginger

1 teaspoon minced garlic

½teaspoon sesame seeds

½teaspoon onion powder

1 tablespoon salt

Directions:

Combine the rice vinegar, oyster sauce, fish sauce, and coconut aminos in a large bowl. Place the short ribs in the marinade and let it sit for 1 hour.

In a separate bowl, mix the pepper flakes, ginger, garlic, onion powder, salt, and sesame seeds. Rub the spice mix into the marinated short ribs.

Place the short ribs on the barbecue grill and cook each side for 5 minutes. Remove the meat from the grill and slice into smaller portions. Serve while hot.

This recipe yields 6 servings.

10.   Low-Carb Vegetarian Pan Pizza

Ingredients:

2 tablespoons psyllium husk powder

4 eggs

1 teaspoon Italian seasoning

3 tablespoons parmesan cheese

3 teaspoons olive oil

Pinch of salt

2 tablespoons freshly-chopped basil leaves

1 cup cheddar cheese, grated

4 tablespoons tomato sauce

Directions:

For the pizza crust batter, combine eggs, psyllium husk, parmesan cheese and salt in a blender and mix well.
Set aside.

Heat the olive oil in a large pan over medium-high flame. Pour half of the pizza crust batter into the pan and let it cook for 2-3 minutes. Flip the pizza crust and cook the remaining side for 2 minutes. Make another pizza crust using the same procedure.

Place both pizza crusts on a baking sheet. Spoon equal portions of tomato sauce, grated cheese and chopped basil on the pizza crust. Bake the pizza in a 225 ° F oven for 5-10 minutes.

This recipe yields 2 servings.

11.   Oven-Baked Rib-eye Steak

Ingredients:

3 medium rib-eye steaks

3 tablespoons butter

1 tablespoon paprika

1 tablespoon garlic powder

Pinch of salt and ground black pepper

Directions:

Rub the rib-eye steaks with salt, pepper, paprika and garlic powder. Place it in a lightly-greased baking dish.

Bake the steaks in a 250 ° F oven for 45 minutes.

Use a cooking thermometer to check for the steak's doneness. If it reaches 120 ° F then the steak is ready.

Remove the steak from the oven and let it stand for 5 minutes.

Heat the butter in a pan over medium flame. Once the oil is hot, place the steaks on the pan and sear each side of the meat for 30-40 seconds. Serve immediately.
This recipe yields 3 servings.

12.   Pan-Fried Chicken Breast with Citrus Sauce

Ingredients:

3 chicken breast halves, skin intact

2 cups kale leaves, washed and stems discarded

½ teaspoon butter

2 tablespoons heavy cream

3 tablespoons olive oil

2 tablespoons organic honey

½teaspoon dried rosemary

1 cup fresh orange juice

Pinch of salt and ground black pepper Directions:

Season the chicken breast with salt and pepper. Place it in a pan over medium-high flame and cook each side for 8-10 minutes. Set aside.

While the chicken breasts are cooking, heat the olive oil in a pan over medium flame. Add in the rosemary, orange juice and honey and simmer for 5-7 minutes. Pour in the heavy cream and cook for 3 minutes. Turn off the heat and set aside.

Place the butter and kale leaves on the same pan where the chicken breast was cooked. Cook the greens for 3-5 minutes or until the leaves wilt.

Transfer the wilted greens on a plate and arrange the chicken breasts on top of it. Pour the orange sauce on top of the dish. Serve immediately.

This recipe yields 3 servings.

13. Flaky Coconut Crusted Shrimp with Tangy Chili Dip

Ingredients:

450 grams shrimps, peeled and deveined

2 tablespoons coconut flour

1 cup dried coconut flakes

2 egg whites

1 red chili, minced

½cup crushed pineapple

1 tablespoon lemon juice

1½ tablespoons white vinegar Pinch of red pepper flakes Directions:

Preheat the oven to 225 ° F and line a baking sheet with parchment paper.

Beat the egg whites until soft white peaks form. Set this aside. Place the coconut flour and coconut flakes in separate bowls.

Dip each shrimp in this order: coconut flour, egg whites then coconut flakes. Arrange the shrimps on the baking sheet until all seafood has been coated. Place the shrimps in the oven and bake for 5 minutes. Turn off the oven

 and arrange the shrimp on a serving platter.

To make the dip, mix together the crushed pineapple, lemon juice, vinegar and pepper flakes. Place the mixture in a sauce bowl and serve alongside the coconut shrimp.

This recipe yields 4 servings.

14.   Crock Pot Leg of Lamb with Fresh Herb Sauce

Ingredients:

900 grams lamb leg

2 tablespoons Dijon mustard

3 garlic cloves, minced

4 fresh thyme sprigs

¼ cup olive oil

1 teaspoon fresh rosemary

1 tablespoon organic honey

6 mint leaves

Pinch of salt and ground black pepper

Directions:

Make 3-4 hollow slices into the lamb leg and place equal amounts of garlic and rosemary into the slits. Place the lamb in the slow cooker and season it with salt, pepper, honey and mustard.

Cover the crock pot and cook the leg on low for 7 hours. After 7 hours, add in the mint leaves and thyme then cook the meat for 1 hour.

Remove the lamb from the pot and slice. Serve hot.

This recipe yields 6 servings.

Chapter 6:
Snack Recipes

Snacking is definitely allowed in the ketogenic diet. Just remember to use organic ingredients such as vegetables, meats and high-fat oils to create healthier versions of your favorite chips, crackers or spreads.

1. Spicy Baked Zucchini Chips

Ingredients:

1 large zucchini, sliced thinly

1 teaspoon paprika

½teaspoon chili powder

3 teaspoons coconut oil

½teaspoon ground white pepper

½teaspoon salt

Directions:

Place the zucchini slices in a colander, sprinkle salt over it and let it stand in the sink for 1 hour. This allows water from the zucchini to drain out completely. Once the water has been completely drained, pat the zucchini slices with a paper towel and set aside.

Line a baking sheet with parchment paper and preheat the oven to 300 ° F. Grease the parchment with a little oil. Arrange the zucchini slices evenly on the baking sheet. Brush some oil on the vegetable slices then sprinkle it salt, pepper, paprika and chili powder.

Place the zucchini in the oven and bake for 30 minutes. Turn off the oven but let the vegetable chips continue cooking for 45 minutes.

This recipe yields 3-4 servings.

2. Garlicky Pork Chips

Ingredients:

200 grams freshly-sliced prosciutto, cut into thin strips

1 teaspoon garlic powder

Directions:

Preheat the oven to 350 ° F and prepare a parchment-lined baking sheet.

Place the prosciutto on the baking sheet. Sprinkle garlic powder on top of the prosciutto. Place the sheet inside the oven and bake for 10-15 minutes. Make sure to keep an eye on the prosciutto to prevent it from burning.

Once the prosciutto is golden brown, remove it from the oven and let it cool on a wire rack. Lightly tap or tear the prosciutto to make chips. Serve immediately.

This recipe yields 3 servings.

3. **Extra Spicy Devilled Eggs**

Ingredients:

8 hard-boiled eggs, peeled

1 tablespoon Dijon mustard

4 tablespoons mayonnaise

1 teaspoon hot sauce
Pinch of paprika

Directions:

Slice each hard-boiled egg in half and scoop out the yolk. Place the yolks in a bowl and set aside the whites.

Add mustard, mayonnaise, hot sauce and paprika to the yolks and mash the ingredients together. Place the yolk mixture in a piping bag. Place 8 egg white halves on a plate. Pipe the yolk mixture beginning from the hollow portion of the egg white moving upwards. Place the other egg white halves on top of the devilled eggs. Serve warm.

This recipe yields 8 servings.

4. **Nutty Spiced Kale Chips**

Ingredients:

2 bunches of kale, washed and stems removed

1 tablespoon honey

2 tablespoons olive oil

½cup lemon juice

½cup almond butter

½cup peanut butter

½tablespoon coconut aminos

½cup apple cider vinegar

1 tablespoon balsamic vinegar

1 red bell pepper, deseeded and chopped

¼cup nutritional yeast

1 teaspoon garlic powder Pinch of salt and black pepper Directions:

Chop the kale into bite-sized pieces and place them on a

layer of paper towels to dry. Set this aside. Preheat the

oven to 200 ° F and line a baking sheet with parchment

paper. Set this aside.

While the kale leaves are drying, place all of the spices, oils, nut butters and vinegars into a food processor. Add in the honey, yeast, bell pepper, lemon juice and coconut aminos. Blend the ingredients until a creamy paste is produced. Season the mixture with salt and pepper.

Pour the nut butter mixture in a large mixing bowl. Add in the kale leaves and toss until the leaves are evenly coated. Arrange the kale leaves on the baking sheet, making sure to not overcrowd it. Place it in the oven and bake the kale for 3 hours or until the leaves are crispy.

This recipe yields 4 servings.

5. **Hot and Spicy Turnip Fries**

Ingredients:

2 turnips, peeled and sliced into thick strips

½teaspoon chili powder

½teaspoon paprika

1 tablespoon olive oil

Pinch of salt and black pepper
Directions:

Preheat the oven to 375 ° F and prepare a parchment-lined baking sheet.

Place the turnip fries in a large bowl and drizzle olive oil on top. Season the vegetable with chili powder, paprika, salt and pepper then toss for an even coating.

Arrange the turnip fries evenly on the baking sheet and place it in the oven. Bake for 25-30 minutes or until the turnip fries become light brown in color. You may also check for the tenderness of the fries by poking them with a skewer.

This recipe yields 4 servings.

6. __Cheesy Baked Sugar Snap Peas__

Ingredients:

4 cups sugar snap peas, washed and drained

2 tablespoons grated parmesan cheese

2 teaspoons olive oil

½ teaspoon garlic powder Pinch of sea salt

Mayonnaise and lemon juice for dipping Directions:

Arrange the snap peas on a baking sheet and drizzle olive oil on top of it. Season the vegetables with salt and garlic powder then sprinkle the grated cheese on top.

Place the snap peas in a 425 ° F oven and bake for 15 minutes. After 15 minutes, flip the snap peas over and continue baking for another 15 minutes.

Arrange the baked snap peas on a plate. Make a mayo and lemon juice dip to complement the flavors of the vegetables. Serve hot.

This recipe yields 2-3 servings.

7. __Bacon and Sausage Knots__

Ingredients:

10 Italian Sausages, sliced into 4

20 bacon strips, halved

2 cups olive oil

20 toothpicks Directions:

Heat the olive oil in a pan over high flame.

Wrap each sausage piece with bacon, covering the sides and the sliced areas. Place toothpicks to secure the bacon around the sausage.

Deep fry the sausages for 4 minutes or until the bacon turns golden brown. Lay the snacks on paper towels to drain any excess oil.

This recipe yields 10 servings.

8. __Crispy Brussels Sprouts with Hot Mayo Sauce__

Ingredients:

4 cups Brussels sprouts, washed and drained
2 teaspoons lemon juice

¾ cup mayonnaise

2 teaspoons hot sauce

3 cups olive oil

Directions:

Slice the Brussels sprouts in quarters and set aside.

Heat the olive oil in a deep frying pan over high flame. Deep fry the vegetables in 6-8 batches. Place the fried vegetables on a layer of paper towels to drain excess oil.

To make the sauce, combine the lemon juice, mayonnaise, hot sauce and salt in a bowl. Whisk until a smooth texture forms.

Arrange the fried Brussels sprouts on a large plate. Drizzle the mayonnaise over the vegetables and lightly toss.

Serve while hot.

This recipe makes 12 servings.

9. <u>Creamy Ham and Asparagus Rollups</u>

Ingredients:

6 large slices of cooked ham

6 asparagus sticks, bottoms trimmed off

3 cups cottage cheese

18 toothpicks Directions:

Boil the asparagus sticks in water for 5 minutes. Once the vegetables are tender, remove them from the heat and drain the water completely.

Lay a slice of ham on the chopping board. Spoon a half cup of cottage cheese on the ham, then place an asparagus stick at the bottom part. Slowly roll the ham upwards. Slice the dish into 3 and secure each portion with a toothpick. Serve immediately.

This recipe yields 6 servings.

10. <u>Celery Sticks with Homemade Nut Butter Dip</u>

Ingredients:

2 cups celery sticks

1 cup almonds, toasted

2 cups macadamia nuts, toasted

1 teaspoon organic honey

¼ teaspoon sea salt ½ teaspoon vanilla Directions:

Place the almonds, macadamia nuts, honey, salt and vanilla in a food processor. Blend the ingredients for 3 minutes. Pour the nut butter in a jar or sauce bowl.

Arrange the celery sticks on a plate. Serve with a side of homemade nut butter.

This recipe yields 3-4 servings.

11.   **Light and Healthy Spinach Crackers**

Ingredients:

150 grams frozen spinach, thawed and drained

¼ cup coconut flour

½ cup grated parmesan cheese 1½ cups almond flour

½cup flaxseed meal

½teaspoon red pepper flakes

½teaspoon cumin powder

¼ cup softened butter ½ teaspoon sea salt Directions:

Boil the spinach leaves and a cup of water in a saucepan for 1 minute. Drain the spinach leaves and use your hand to squeeze out any excess liquid from the leaves. Place the spinach in a food processor and blend for 30 seconds. Set aside.

Combine the coconut flour, almond flour, parmesan cheese and softened butter in a bowl. Mix well. Season the dry ingredients with salt, cumin and red pepper flakes.

Add in the ground spinach and mix until a soft dough forms. Place the dough in between two sheets of wax paper and use a rolling pin to flatten it. Transfer the flattened dough on a parchment-lined baking sheet and continue rolling it to the sides of the sheet.

Slice the dough into squares and place it in the oven. Bake it for 30 minutes at 250 ° F.

This recipe yields 8 servings.

12.   **Yummy Bacon and Egg Bites**

Ingredients:

2 medium hard-boiled egg, peeled

1 tablespoon mayonnaise

2 tablespoons softened butter

2 bacon slices, cooked

Pinch of salt and ground black pepper

Directions:

Chop the cooked bacon into small pieces and set aside.

Combine the hard-boiled eggs, butter and mayonnaise in a bowl. Mash the ingredients together and season it with salt and pepper. Form the mixture into 3 balls and roll it into the chopped bacon. Serve immediately.

This recipe yields 3 servings.

13.   **Baked Coconut Crisps**

Ingredients:

4 cups unsweetened coconut flakes

1 teaspoon cinnamon

2 tablespoons Erythritol

1 teaspoon vanilla extract
4 tablespoons coconut oil, melted

Pinch of sea salt

Directions:

Preheat the oven to 350 ° F and prepare a parchment-lined baking sheet.

Place the coconut flakes in a large bowl. Add in the cinnamon, Erythritol, vanilla, coconut oil and salt. Toss the ingredients together.

Transfer the coconut flakes on the baking sheet and place it in the oven. Bake for 5 minutes or until the flakes turn light brown. Remove the coconut from the oven and let it cool on a wire rack.

This recipe yields 8 servings.

14.   **Low-Carb Caprese Salad Sticks**

Ingredients:

4 cups small mozzarella balls

1 cup mixed olives, pitted

4 cups cherry tomatoes

4 tablespoons fresh basil leaves

4 tablespoons pesto sauce

1 teaspoon olive oil

4 skewers Directions:

In a small bowl, combine the mozzarella and pesto. Mix well until the mozzarella is evenly coated.

Get a skewer and pierce a tomato through it, followed by a mozzarella ball, an olive and a basil leaf. Do another row of the same ingredients. Create 3 more Caprese salad sticks then arrange them on a plate. Drizzle olive oil on top and serve.

This recipe yields 4 servings.

Chapter 7:
Dessert Recipes

C ombining small amounts of fruit, chocolate, natural sweeteners, oils and organic flours helps create nutritious and delectable ketogenic-friendly desserts. But do remember that small amounts of dessert yield better results, especially around the waistline.

1. Freezer–Friendly Chocolate Pudding

Ingredients:

4 tablespoons cocoa powder

2 cups full fat coconut milk

1 ½ teaspoon stevia powder extract

3 tablespoons water

2 tablespoons powdered gelatin

Directions:

Place the cocoa powder, stevia and coconut milk in a saucepan over medium heat. Slowly mix until the cocoa is dissolved.

In a separate bowl, blend the gelatin and water until the gelatin dissolves. Pour the gelatin mixture into the cocoa mixture and mix thoroughly.

Once the pudding mixture starts to heat up, turn off the stove. Pour the pudding mixture into 4 ramekins or pudding cups and place them in the freezer to set.

This recipe yields 4 servings.

2. Luscious Coconut Brownies

Ingredients:

1 cup cocoa powder

2 teaspoons stevia powder extract

2 large eggs

1 cup almond flour

½cup shredded coconut

1 teaspoon vanilla

½teaspoon baking soda

½cup chopped almonds

½cup coconut milk

1 cup coconut oil, melted

Directions:

Prepare a square baking pan by brushing it lightly with olive oil. Preheat the oven to 350 ° F.

Place the baking soda, coconut and almond flour in a mixing bowl and blend thoroughly. In another bowl, whisk together eggs, vanilla, stevia, cocoa powder, coconut milk and coconut oil. Combine both mixtures together then gradually fold in the almonds.

Pour the brownie mixture into the pan and bake in the oven for 30 minutes. Let the brownies cool before slicing it into 9 squares.
This recipe yields 9 servings.

3. **Chocolate Almond Squares**

Ingredients:

120 grams dark chocolate chips

1 cup shredded coconut

1 cup almond flour

3 tablespoons coconut oil

1 ½ cups almond butter

¾ cup coconut sugar Directions:

Heat the almond butter and 2 tablespoons of the coconut oil in a saucepan over medium-low flame. Once the ingredients have melted, turn off the heat. Fold in the almond flour, coconut sugar and shredded coconut into the saucepan and mix well.

Pour the almond mixture into a square-sized baking pan and set aside.

Heat the chocolate chips and remaining coconut oil in a saucepan over medium flame until the chocolate melts.
Mix well.

Pour the melted chocolate mixture on top of the almond mixture, making sure that the top of the dessert is evenly-coated. Refrigerate for 2 hours then slice the dessert into 20 almond squares.

This recipe yields 10 servings.

4. Chewy Chocolate Zucchini Brownies

Ingredients:

1 cup gluten free semi-sweet chocolate chips

1 ½ cups shredded zucchini, drained

1 cup almond butter

1 large egg

1 teaspoon cinnamon

1 teaspoon baking soda

½ cup organic honey Directions:

Preheat the oven to 350 ° F and lightly grease a 9x9 baking pan.

Combine the zucchini, chocolate chips, egg, almond butter, honey, baking soda and cinnamon in a mixing bowl. Pour the mixture into the baking pan.

Bake the brownies for 45 minutes. Slice into squares and serve.

This recipe yields 9 servings.

5. Coconut Pudding with Fresh Berries

Ingredients:

2 cups full-fat coconut milk

1 cup fresh strawberries, stems removed

½ cup blueberries
½ tablespoon stevia

½teaspoon vanilla

3 tablespoons flaxseeds

Directions:

Place the coconut milk, strawberries, mangoes, stevia, vanilla and flaxseeds in a blender and pulse until the ingredients are mixed well.

Pour the mixture into 2 bowls and place it in the freezer for 1 hour. Serve chilled.

This recipe yields 2 servings.

6. Almond Coconut Fat Bombs

Ingredients:

2 tablespoons almond butter

1 cup softened cold-pressed coconut oil

3 tablespoons unsweetened cocoa powder

2 tablespoons organic honey

1 teaspoon vanilla

½ teaspoon sea salt

1 cup shredded coconut

Directions:

Place the almond butter, coconut oil, cocoa powder, honey, vanilla and sea salt in a food processor and mix until smooth and creamy.

Form the mixture into 16 candy balls. Roll each ball into the shredded coconut and place on a parchment-lined sheet. Refrigerate the candies for 1 hour then transfer them in an airtight container.

This recipe yields 8 servings.

7. Frozen Watermelon Creamsicles

Ingredients:

2 cups watermelon chunks, deseeded

1 ¾ cups full-fat coconut milk

1 teaspoon vanilla

1 tablespoon organic honey

Directions:

Puree the watermelon in a food processor and pour it into a bowl, making sure to discard seeds. Place the fruit puree back into the food processor then pour in the honey, vanilla and coconut milk. Process until the mixture becomes smooth and creamy.

Pour the watermelon mixture into 4 molds and place popsicle sticks through the dessert. Place the popsicles in the freezer for 4-5 hours.

This recipe yields 4 servings.

8. Low-Carb Cinnamon Pumpkin Blondie

Ingredients:

1 teaspoon cinnamon
1 cup canned pumpkin puree

½cup organic honey

1 cup almond butter

1 teaspoon baking soda

1 tablespoon melted coconut oil

1 egg

1 teaspoon vanilla extract Directions:

Place the pumpkin puree in a mixing bowl. Add in the cinnamon, honey, almond butter, baking soda, coconut oil, egg and vanilla extract. Mix well.

Pour the batter into a square 8x8 baking pan. Bake the dish in a preheated 350 ° F oven for 30 minutes. Slice into squares and serve. This recipe yields 9 servings.

9. **Watermelon & Cucumber Sorbet**

Ingredients:

1 ½ cup diced cucumber meat

4 cups watermelon chunks, deseeded

2 tablespoons lime juice

2 tablespoons Erythritol

1 cup crushed ice

Directions:

Combine the cucumber, watermelon, lime juice, Erythritol and ice in a blender and mix for 15-20 seconds. Pour the mixture into a stainless bowl and freeze for 2 hours.

Take out the sorbet from the freezer and let it stand for 5 minutes. Scoop the sorbet into individual cups and serve.

This recipe yields 3 servings.

10. **Heavenly Chocolate Bacon Strips**

Ingredients:

16 bacon slices (thin slices)

2 tablespoons Erythritol

1 tablespoon coconut oil

1 teaspoon maple syrup

1 cup dark chocolate chips

Pinch of cinnamon powder

Directions:

Preheat the oven to 275 ° F and line a baking sheet with parchment paper.

In a small bowl combine the cinnamon powder and Erythritol. Sprinkle the mixture on both sides of the bacon.

Arrange the bacon on the baking sheet and bake it in the oven for 60 minutes. The bacon should be crisp and golden brown in color. To make the chocolate coating, melt the chocolate chips with the coconut oil and maple syrup using a double boiler. Stir until the chocolate melts and is warm to the touch.

Take out the bacon from the oven and let it cool for 5 minutes. Use a spoon to coat the bacon with the melted chocolate. Let the chocolate-covered bacon harden on a baking sheet. Place the bacon strips in the fridge.

This recipe yields 8 servings.

11. Vanilla Meringue Bites

Ingredients:

½teaspoon vanilla extract

½teaspoon apple cider vinegar

1 ½ tablespoon Erythritol

4 egg whites Directions:

Preheat the oven to 275 ° F and prepare a parchment-lined cookie sheet.

Whisk the egg whites using an electric mixer and place it on medium-low speed for 2 minutes. Once the eggs become foamy, gradually mix in the apple cider vinegar, vanilla and Erythritol. Beat the whites until glossy white peaks form.

Place the meringue mixture in a piping bag and pipe 24 small mounds on the cookie sheet. Bake the meringue in the oven for 15 minutes then lower the temperature to 200 ° F. Continue baking the dessert for 1 hour. Let it cool in room temperature before serving.

This recipe yields 6 servings.

12. High Fiber Blueberry Milkshake

Ingredients:

1 cup fresh blueberries

1 cup coconut milk

½ cup almond milk

2 tablespoons melted coconut oil

1 ½ tablespoons chia seeds

2 drops liquid stevia

1 teaspoon vanilla extract

½ cup crushed ice Directions:

Pour the coconut milk, almond milk, vanilla and coconut oil into a blender and pulse. Add in the blueberries, chia seeds, stevia and ice and process until smooth. Pour the milkshake into individual glasses and serve.

This recipe yields 2 servings.

13.   Chocolate Peppermint Bark

Ingredients:

4 tablespoons coconut oil, melted

½ teaspoon peppermint extract

2 tablespoons unsweetened cocoa powder
 2 tablespoons Erythritol

2 tablespoons heavy cream

2 tablespoons toasted almonds, chopped

Pinch of sea salt

Directions:

Combine coconut oil, peppermint extract, cocoa powder, Erythritol, salt and toasted almonds in a bowl. Fold in the heavy cream and mix until the texture becomes silky.

Pour the chocolate mixture in a lined baking pan then place it in the freezer for 2-3 hours.

Break apart the chocolate bark into bite-sized pieces. Serve frozen.

This recipe yields 4 servings.

14.   Mini Strawberry Cheesecake Balls

Ingredients:

¾ cups softened cream cheese

½ cup frozen strawberries, thawed

1 tablespoon almond extract ¼ cup butter

2 tablespoons Erythritol

1 cup almond flour Directions:

Let the butter and cream cheese melt in a bowl at room temperature for 45 minutes. Once melted, place the ingredients in a food processor.

Add in the almond extract, Erythritol and strawberries. Mix the ingredients until the mixture turns creamy.

Use a spoon to make small round balls from the cheesecake mixture. Roll it on a plate with almond flour then place it in a small cupcake liner.

Freeze the dessert for 2 hours. Serve chilled.

This recipe yields 10-12 servings.

Conclusion

Thank you again for downloading this book!

I hope this book was able to encourage you to adopt an effective ketogenic meal planning system based on the low-carbohydrate recipes that were shown in the preceding chapters

Moreover, I hope that you will regularly practice a ketogenic lifestyle as this will not only help you achieve a healthy weight, but will also create a positively life-changing balance between the mind, body, and soul.

The next step is to try out more ketogenic recipes from this book and create a meal plan that will best suit your lifestyle and health goals.

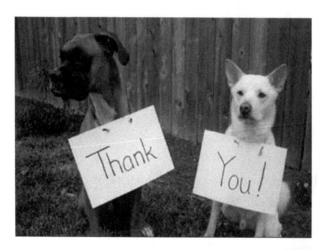

Finally, if you enjoyed this book, then I'd like to ask you for a favor, would you be kind enough to leave a review for this book on Amazon? It'd be greatly appreciated!

Click here to leave a review for this book on Amazon!

or go to http://amzn.to/1YwE9N1

Thank you and good luck!

Preview Of 'Running Guide for Beginners: How to Start Running for Weight Loss and Increase Endurance'

Chapter 1 – Benefits of Running

For most people, running does not seem to be an effective way to lose weight. Although going to the gym and lifting heavy dumbbells can really help in toning your muscles, it doesn't mean that jogging a few laps around the park is useless.

In fact, running will not just strengthen your leg muscles; it will also improve your bone density, relieve stress, and even fortify your immune system. Can you believe that a *simple physical exercise* can do so much? If not, check out these other compelling reasons why should start running today!

1. Keeps depression at bay

When you are depressed, it is understandable that you will feel too lazy or weak to run outdoors. However, it is highly recommended that you try running because it'll definitely remove the blues out of your system.

Click here to check out the rest of "Running Guide for Begineers" on Amazon.

Or go to: amzn.to/2oHlVsr
Check Out Other Books

Below you'll find some of other popular books that are popular on Amazon and Kindle as well. Simply click on the links below to check them out.

Running Guide for Beginners: How to Start Running for Weight Loss and Increase Endurance
- *Chris Douglas*

STRETCHING: Pre and Post Running Stretching Exercises
- *Chris Douglas*

Meditation and Mindfulness for Beginners: Easy, Simple and Practical Steps to Relieve Stress, Anxiety and Achieve Peace and Happiness
- *Chris Douglas*

KETO CHAFFLE

200 Easy Chaffle recipes for fast fat burning, weight loss and metabolism boost, including keto snacks. Delicious keto desserts cookbook to start your keto diet, right now!

Table of Contents

MEDICAL DISCLAIMER

This book details the author's personal experiences and opinions about right- brained learning. The author is not licensed as an educational consultant, teacher, psychologist, or psychiatrist.

The author and publisher are providing this book and its contents on an "as is" basis and make no representations or warranties of any kind with respect to this book or its contents. The author and publisher disclaim all such representations and warranties, including for example warranties of merchantability and educational or medical advice for a particular purpose. In addition, the author and publisher do not represent or warrant that the information accessible via this book is accurate, complete or current.

Except as specifically stated in this book, neither the author or publisher, nor any authors, contributors, or other representatives will be liable for damages arising out of or in connection with the use of this book. This is a comprehensive limitation of liability that applies to all damages of any kind, including (without limitation) compensatory; direct, indirect or consequential damages; loss of data, income or profit; loss of or damage to property and claims of third parties.

You understand that this book is not intended as a substitute for consultation with a licensed medical, educational, legal or accounting professional. Before you begin any change in your lifestyle in any way, you will consult a licensed professional to ensure that you are doing what's best for your situation.

This book provides content related to educational, medical, and psychological topics. As such, the use of this book implies your acceptance of this disclaimer.

THE KETOGENIC DIET

The Ketogenic Diet, or as it is regularly known, "Keto Diet," was initially used to control seizures among individuals who endured epilepsy. It is not some new pattern or "in" thing. The diet has been around since the mid-1900's and has entrenched itself in the studies of nourishment and medication.

The Ketogenic Diet comprises of eating high segments of fat while downplaying starch utilization with a moderate measure of protein added to support bulk. A keto diet's essential point is to have your body depend on fats for vitality in a state called ketosis.

A ketogenic diet is a low carb, a high-fat diet that transforms your body into a fat-burning machine. At the point when insulin - the fat putting away hormone - levels drop, you will feel the distinction of an ideal body. Keto has many weight reduction, wellbeing, and execution benefits for type 2 diabetes, epilepsy, PCOS, metabolic disorder, pulse, cholesterol, mental concentration, and various immune system infections.

Keto confines your admission of sugar and dull foods, similar to pasta and bread. Rather, you will eat tasty, genuine food with a particular protein, sound fats, and vegetables for supplements. K contains all that you need - what to eat, what to stay away from, and precisely how to do it.

What is Ketosis, and how does a Keto Diet realize it?

Ketosis happens when your body stops to depend on sugars as fuel. Your liver starts to change over the fat put away in your body into fatty acids and ketone bodies. These ketone bodies, at that point, supplant glucose as the body's vitality source.

Moving from sugars or glucose for vitality to fat as the bodies essential fuel source is valuable in the way that;

- You accomplish a more drawn out enduring, continued vitality.

- You have more honed fixation and mental core interest.

- You do not require progressively visit refeeds, as your body's vitality source is presently any longer enduring and consistent.

Contradicted to the short spikes, up's and downs, and inevitable crashes that you get with straightforward sugars and even that of complex starches.

Numerous tip-top games individuals that contend in occasions of continuance have changed this one explanation too along these lines of eating. However, it is by all account, not the only explanation.

A ketogenic diet places the body in a condition of ketosis, where the essential fuel for the body is a separated result of fat called ketone bodies. Ketosis can happen through the decrease of sugars in the eating regimen or through fasting (or through taking an outer ketone-creating item). The liver produces ketone bodies by separating unsaturated fats, either from muscle to fat ratio or the fat that we eat.

This is rather than the body's fuel source when not in ketosis: sugars, which the body separates into glucose.

It is imperative to take note that there is a distinction between consuming dietary fat for fuel and getting the body to use put away fat.
The ketogenic diet is such a low-carbohydrate, a high-fat eating routine that offers numerous similitudes with the Atkins and low-carb eats fewer carbs.

It includes radically lessening sugar admission and supplanting it with fat. This decrease in carbs places the body into a metabolic condition called ketosis. At the point when this happened, the body turns out to be unfathomably productive at consuming fat for vitality. It likewise converts fat into ketones in the liver, which can supply energy for the cerebrum.
Ketogenic diets can cause large decreases in glucose and insulin intake or levels. These have various medical advantages.
A regular low starch diet may mainly concentrate on restricting sugar with liberal measures of different sustenance's, without a particular accentuation on fats. It is anything but challenging to generally eat meats and some other non-starch nourishments for a low sugar diet, and not get into ketosis.

So what is unique? The ketogenic diet goes beyond and limits protein too to accomplish ketosis. A ketogenic diet is contained:

· 65 – 80% of calories from fat

· 10 – 15% of calories from proteins (0.5 gram per lb. of fit weight)
· 5 – 10% calories from starches.

3

Various Types of Ketogenic Diets

There are a few renditions of the ketogenic diet, including:

··**The standard ketogenic diet (SKD):**Thus a low-carb, moderate-protein, and high-fat diet. It contains 75% fat, 20% protein, and just 5% carbs (1).

··**The cyclical ketogenic diet (CKD):**This diet includes times of higher-carb refeeds. For example, five ketogenic days pursued by two high-carb days.

··**The targeted ketogenic diet (TKD):**This diet enables you to include and target some diets carbs with exercises.
·

•**High-protein ketogenic diet**: This is like an example of a standard keto diet, yet it includes more protein. The proportion is regularly 60% fat, 35%

protein, and 5% carbs.

· Nonetheless, just the standard and high-protein ketogenic diets have been examined widely. Repetitive or focused on ketogenic diets are further developed strategies and utilized by muscle heads or competitors.

Other Health Benefits of Keto

The ketogenic diet started as a device for treating neurological illnesses, for example, epilepsy.
Keto diet has benefits for a wide range of wellbeing conditions:

- **Heart infection**: The ketogenic diet can improve hazard components like a muscle to fat ratio. HDL cholesterol levels, circulatory strain, and glucose.

- **Alzheimer's ailment:** The keto diet may lessen the side effects of Alzheimer's sickness and how to moderate its movement.

- **Parkinson's ailment:** One investigation found that the diet improved the side effects of Parkinson's illness.

- **Polycystic ovary disorder:** The ketogenic diet plan or routine can help decrease insulin levels, which may assume a vital job in polycystic ovary disorder.

- **Brain wounds:** One creature concentrate found that the diet could diminish blackouts and help recuperation after cerebrum damage.

- **Acne:** This lowers insulin levels, and eating less sugar, or handled sustenance may help improve skin break out.

Instructions to Eat Keto

In a perfect world, a keto diet ought to be gathered with entire and nutritious sustenance that does not cause inflammation. This implies the 5-10% of the sugars would be from vegetables, nuts, and seeds as opposed to another wellspring of starch.

On a keto-type diet, the plate should comprise of, for the most part, non-bland vegetables, a sensible segment of meat (around 3 ounces), and a liberal measure of good fats. The fats can be nuts, seeds, olive oil, avocados, avocado oil, fed fat or bacon, grass-bolstered spread, MCT oil, or a topping like a sound mayo produced using these.

When an individual is keto-adjusted, the hunger is regularly directed. Instead of inclination denied, it is reasonable to feel less hungry in general and customarily slanted to abandon eating for 12 hours medium-term. This type of broadened fasting may give some additional medical advantages also.

Nourishments to Avoid

Any food that has excess carbohydrates ought to be restricted.

Here is a rundown of nourishments that should be diminished or wiped out on a ketogenic diet:

- **Sugary nourishments:** Soda, organic product juice, smoothies, cake, dessert, sweet, and so on.

- **Grains or starches:** Wheat-based items, oat, pasta, rice, and so on.

- **Fruit:**All organic products, except for little parts of berries like strawberries.

- **Beans or vegetables:**Chickpeas, Peas, kidney beans, lentils, and so forth.

- **Root vegetables and tubers:**carrot, sweet potatoes, Potatoes, parsnips, and so forth.

- **Low fat or diet items:**These are exceptionally handled and regularly high in carbs.

- **Some fixings or sauces:**These frequently contain sugar and undesirable fat.

- **Unhealthy fats:**Limit your admission of prepared vegetable oils, mayonnaise, and so on.

- **Alcohol:**Due to their high carb content, numerous mixed refreshments can toss you out of ketosis.

- **Sugar diet sustenance:**These are frequently high in sugar alcohols, which can influence ketone levels sometimes. This sustenance's likewise will, in general, be profoundly handled.

Nourishments to Eat

You should base most of your suppers around this sustenance:

- Meat: Red meat, chicken, steak, ham, sausage, bacon, and turkey.

- **Fatty fish:**Example such as salmon, trout, fish, and mackerel.

- **Eggs:**Look to fed or omega-3 entire eggs.

- **Butter and cream:**Look for grass-bolstered when conceivable.

- **Cheese:**Unprocessed (cheddar, goat, cream, blue, or mozzarella).

- **Nuts and seeds:**Examples like Almonds, pecans, flax seeds, pumpkin seeds, chia seeds, and so on.

- **Healthy oils:**Primarily additional virgin olive oil, and avocado oil.

- **Avocados:**Whole avocados or crisply made guacamole.

- **Low-carb vegetable:**Most onions, green vegetables, tomatoes, onions, peppers, and so on.

- **Condiments:**You can utilize pepper, salt and different sound herbs and flavors.

- It is ideal for putting together your diet for the most part concerning entire, single-fixing sustenance.

The most effective method to get into Ketosis

Ketosis is accomplished by taking out sugar, sugary natural product, grains, bread, pasta, root vegetables and supplanting them with non-boring vegetables, meats, eggs, full creams, solid oils, eating on high fat – low carb nuts, for example, Brazil Nuts, and macadamias, and an entire bundle of other high fat low carb foods.

The Keto Diet is definitely not exhausting. When you overcome your dependence on sugars, you will be eating like Royalty.

Be that as it may, ketosis just happens once the body never again has the way to utilize sugars or all the more distinctly glucose as its first decision vitality source. Only one huge portion of carbs will see you spiking your insulin, handling glucose, and stopping to be in ketosis. (Your body will consistently utilize carbs first).

7

Along these lines, it is basic that you screen what you eat and keep your carb admission beneath 30grams or less of net carbs (net carbs = all out carbs − fiber carbs) every day to stay in ketosis.

A few people should limit their carbs to even not as much as that due to:

- Size

- Gender

- And plain old hereditary qualities

If you can oversee 15 grams of carbs a day, you will see yourself in ketosis in a matter of moments. This low carb admission is the fundamental contrast between simply any low carb diet and a ketogenic diet.

WHY YOU SHOULD TRY A KETOGENIC DIET

The fit human body is 74% fat and 26% protein (separated by calories). Fats are an auxiliary piece of each human cell and are the favored fuel wellspring of the mitochondria, the vitality burning units of every phone. A hatchling normally utilizes ketones previously and the following birth. This post will give you the data you need concerning why you ought to consider a ketogenic diet.

Aggravation is the stem of everything being equal. One inquiry or protest is the reason, wouldn't I be able to eat "ordinary?" Sure, there are individuals who can eat potatoes and rice and pasta and not be overweight, BUT this does not mean they are sound. I have had a bunch of customers who were female, 115 pounds, and had exceptionally high glucose levels and must be put on insulin. Not exclusively should diabetics and individuals who need to get more fit farthest point starch admission, everybody should.

We are all, in a transformative sense, inclined to get diabetic. Therefore, I need to step you through how fat is put away; however, more critically, this is the manner by which we become in danger for diabetes and coronary illness:

1. After you eat abundance starches, the blood glucose remains higher longer in light of the fact that the glucose cannot make it into the cells of the muscles. This harmful degree of glucose resembles tar in the circulatory system stopping up courses, authoritative with proteins to frame harming AGEs (Advanced Glycated End-items), and causing aggravation. This elevated level of glucose makes triglycerides go up, expanding your hazard for coronary illness.

2. Starch and sugar are put away as fat (recollect starch is simply glucose particles snared together in a long chain; the stomach related track separates it into glucose... so a sugary and a starch diet is something very similar!). Since the muscle cells are not getting glycogen (since they essentially have an outside layer over the cells and are considered "safe"), and since insulin stops the generation of the fat-burning compound lipase, presently, you cannot burn STORED fat! So exercise all you need, on the off chance that you keep on eating cereal before your exercises, you will never be a fat-burner, you will stay a sugar-burner, and you keep on getting fatter until in the end, those fat cells become safe as well.

3. On the off chance that that is not awful enough, I have even more terrible news... Insulin levels keep on remaining high longer in light of the fact that the pancreas erroneously accepts "if a little isn't working, more is

better." NOT GOOD. Insulin is dangerous at elevated levels, causing cell harm, tumors, plaque development in the supply routes (which is the reason diabetics have such a lot of coronary illness) just as numerous other aggravation issues, for example, nerve harm and agony in the furthest points. Starch and sugar decimate nerve tissue, causing shivering and retinopathy, which makes you lose your vision.

4. Apologies, yet I have even more awful news... Our phones become so harmed after an existence of oat and skim milk for breakfast that not exclusively does insulin opposition square glucose from entering muscle cells; the hull we have shaped over our phones additionally squares amino acids from entering. Amino acids are the structure obstructs for our muscles that are found in protein. So now, you cannot keep up your muscles. What's more, if that is not awful enough, our muscles become savages in light of the fact that your body believes there is insufficient put-away sugar in the phones, so they send signs to begin to expend significant muscles to make more glucose (sugar)! You get fatter, and you lose muscle.

5.Rather than feeling fiery after you eat, you are worn out, and you pine for more starches, and since you have less muscle, practice is getting too darn troublesome, and the dismal cycle proceeds.

6. There is much progressively terrible news... thyroid issues likewise happens as well. At the point when your liver becomes insulin safe, it cannot change over thyroid hormone T4 into the T3, so you get those unexplained "thyroid issues," which keep on bringing down your vitality and digestion.

WHAT IS A CHAFFLE?

A Chaffle is a waffle yet made with a cheddar base. Essentially, it has destroyed cheddar and an egg blend. Occasionally for progressively fluffier recipes, it is a cream cheddar base rather than destroyed cheddar. It is the stylish new keto-accommodating bread since its low in carbs, and it will not spike your insulin levels, causing fat stockpiling.

The rudiments are some combo of egg and cheddar; however, from here, you can riff like frantic. You can utilize an assortment of cheeses, including cream cheddar, parmesan cheddar, and so forth. Some include almond flour and flaxseed and preparing powder, and others do not.

The fundamental formula for a Chaffle contains cheddar, almond flour, and an egg. You combine the ingredients in a bowl and pour it over your waffle creator. Waffle creators are most likely on the ascent right now after the Chaffle formula detonated a few days ago prior. I was somewhat doubtful from the start thinking there was no chance this would turn out in the wake of combining everything and pouring the hitter over the waffle. I was expecting one tremendous major chaos. Make a point to splash the waffle producer truly well. The waffle ended up extraordinary, and it was firm outwardly and delicate in the center.

WHAT DO I NEED TO MAKE A CHAFFLE?

• 1 enormous egg

• 1/2 c. Cheddar – I utilized Happy Farms brand from Aldi

• 2 tablespoons of almond flour

HOW TO MAKE A CHAFFLE?

Everybody is going looney tunes, asking, "How would I make these?" This is the arrangement the fundamental formula on what and how. The essential formula incorporates destroyed cheddar and an egg; however, there are huge amounts of add-ins you can use to change the flavor! You will make a straightforward Chaffle hitter and cook it in a waffle creator!

To make a Chaffle formula, you will combine a couple of ingredients and cook it in a waffle creator to make a magnum opus everybody will cherish!

1. Preheat your waffle creator in the event that it requires preheating.

2. Whisk together the egg, cheddar, almond flour, and preparing the soft drink in a bowl until all-around joined.

3. Spray the waffle creator with a cooking splash and pour the Chaffle player over the waffle producer. Close and let the waffle for 3 to 4 minutes. My waffle creator has its own programmed clock setting.

4. Take the waffle out of the waffle press and appreciate it.

THE TYPE OF WAFFLE MAKER NEEDED TO MAKE A CHAFFLE

The vast majority truly prefers to utilize a Dash Mini Waffle Maker; however, you can utilize any waffle producer you have. There is a wide range of waffle producers. Truth be told, you most likely have one in the rear of your kitchen cupboards that you have not utilized in a very long time. The vast majority who do not have a waffle producer may even discover one at a Goodwill or Salvation Army. There is no lack of these convenient kitchen devices in these recycled stores.

THE 4 DIFFERENT TYPES OF BASIC KETO CHAFFLE RECIPES

Keto Chaffle Recipes eBook Cookbook comprises sweet and appetizing keto recipes for each flavor palette.

- Basic Chaffle Recipes

- Savory Chaffle Recipes

- Sweet Chaffle Recipes

- Chaffle Cake Recipes

GUIDELINES ON HOW TO MAKE THE BEST CHAFFLES

1.Patience. That is the best tip. They don't take long, yet in the event that you need a fresh keto waffle, you are simply must be somewhat patient and let it take the 5-7 minutes that it takes to fresh up. Exactly when you believe it has finished? Allow it one more moment or two. Try not to surge.

2. Layering. In case you are making a Chaffle with cheddar, the best approach to do this is to layer cheddar at the base, pour in a tablespoon or so of egg, and afterward top with cheddar once more. It is the firm cheddar on the base and top that will make them fresh.

3. Shallow waffles. In the event that you need fresh waffles, the shallower the waffle iron, the simpler/quicker it is too fresh up the Chaffle.

4. No overloading. Stuffed Chaffle producers... well, they flood obviously. Which makes tremendous wreckage! So if all else fails, under fill as opposed to packing. Close to 1/4 cup of TOTAL ingredients one after another.

5.Squeeze it. I have known about others utilizing press bottles so they can get only a little egg into the mini waffle creator.

6. Easy cleanup. I like to utilize a wet paper towel when the waffle iron is warm, to make cleanup simple. Not hot, however, clearly! Simply warm.

7.Brush it. I have discovered toothbrush functions admirably to clean between the waffle iron teeth. You can likewise attempt this wipe cleaner, which I additionally use to clean the little territory on the edge of my Instant Pot.

8. No looking. I can let you know from LOTS of individual experience, that opening the waffle iron at regular intervals "just to check" does not help the Chaffle cook any quicker. Your most logical option is to not by any means open it for 4-5 minutes.

9. No steaming. In case you are utilizing the Dash mini, the little blue light goes out when it is generally cooked, yet above all, the Chaffle quits steaming to such an extent. That is a decent sign that it has finished.

10.Get hot. Hold up until the waffle iron is hot before you include ingredients, and they're significantly less inclined to stick and much simpler to tidy up.

11. Mat it. OK, so about that flood. I do find that it transpires more regularly than I might want! One thing that has made cleanup simpler for me has been to put a silicone trivet underneath.

12. Slice or shred. I realize most recipes out there recommend destroyed cheddar, yet I have better karma with the most slender cut of cheddar I can purchase. I discover it crisps significantly quicker.

13. Not-so-eggy. In the event that you discover your Chaffle too eggy, use egg white rather than the entire egg.

14. Not-so-gooey. On the off chance that you need them to taste less gooey, attempt mozzarella cheddar.

15. Crispy Cooling. Permit the Chaffle to cool before eating. They get crisper as they cool, so do whatever it takes not to stuff the hot Chaffle into your mouth immediately.

16. Make parts. Make enough to share, and everybody will need them, regardless of whether they are keto or not.

HOW TO CALCULATE NUTRITIONAL VALUES

Keto Calculator to set up your ketogenic macronutrient proportions.

It calculates keto macros in grams and rates to base your ketogenic diet around. Your center (for the principal month at any rate) ought to be on your calculated keto macros. More so, macronutrients than everyday calorie consumption.

KETO MACROS FOR WEIGHT LOSS AND MUSCLE GAIN

The full keto scale-adding machine is movable to deliver various outcomes relying upon your ketogenic diet objectives, for example, weight reduction, upkeep, or muscle gain.

Enter your present load in pounds or kilograms into the Keto Macro Calculator.

At that point, add your muscle versus fat ratio to build up your day-by-day macros.

In case you are uncertain of your muscle versus fat ratio and realize that you are overweight, simply put in 45%.

The most significant thing for those starting the Ketogenic Diet is not adding up to calories devoured (to begin with); it is your disposal of starches and adhering to your macros from the keto adding machine.

By staying with your calculated keto large scale proportions of (roughly) 70% Fat, 25% Protein, and 5% (close to 30gram) Carbohydrates. It has been demonstrated craving will become smothered normally.

Estimating Body Fat for Accurate Keto Macros

You can gauge muscle versus fat "at home" with skin fold estimations. In the event that you need to quantify your skin folds, you will require some reasonable skin crease calipers that you can arrive at.

In the event that you are well overweight and for effortlessness, simply put 45 into the Keto Calculator for your Body Fat Measurement. The subsequently calculated keto macros will be ideal for you.

Follow your macros from the keto number cruncher, and you will see an emotional misfortune in weight.

Ascertaining Calories and Nutrients in Meals

1). Ascertaining Calories and Nutrients in Single Ingredient Meals:

It is not constantly achievable to calculate nourishment data for the entirety of your recipes, yet having data for a portion of your dinners is superior to having nothing by any stretch of the imagination. Ascertaining sustenance data for increasingly standard recipes is an extraordinary spot to begin.

We trust you locate the enclosed proposals on the most proficient method to calculate calorie and supplement data in three situations accommodating:

1). Single Ingredient Meals

2). Recipes and Mixed Dishes

3). Full Meals

For instance, if you need to realize the calorie substance of 2 cups of a food thing, alter the numerical incentive in the segment titled "cup" to 2.

Other unit transformations may occasionally be vital if the unit of intrigue is not an accessible alternative. If you need to realize the calorie substance of 8 oz. of a food thing, yet just the incentive for 100 grams is accessible, at that point, you should change the numerical incentive in the section titled 'esteem per 100 grams' to 3.37.

1 oz. = 30.5 grams

8 oz. = 244 grams (8 x 30.5 grams)

244 grams/100 grams = 2.44 (so you would require 2.44 occasions the 100-gram esteem)

1.A valuable transformation apparatus is required.

2.   Calorie data is the subsequent column and is titled "Vitality." Other nutrients ordinarily announced are in the lines quickly following protein, all-out fat, starch, and absolute dietary fiber. Sodium is in the segment titled "Minerals," and immersed fat, unsaturated fat, and cholesterol are situated in the area titled "Lipids."

Calories, nutrients, and loads showed for every food are for the eatable bit of food (for instance – without bones, and so forth.)

2). Computing calories for recipes and mixed dishes:

A great deal of the foods we eat has more than one ingredient. For instance, a chicken bosom is occasionally arranged plain and may incorporate some kind of fat utilized during cooking, a sauce included thereafter, or different ingredients. Multi-ingredient recipes can be calculated by entering information for every individual ingredient into an MS Excel spreadsheet that has been set up for this reason. The spreadsheet gives you a choice to list what number of servings the formula makes and will calculate the calories and nutrients per serving. Follow the means beneath to calculate the sustenance data for a multi-ingredient food or formula.

1. Type the names and measures of every ingredient into the spreadsheet.

2. Determine calories and nutrients for every individual ingredient in the right amount, as depicted previously.

3. Enter the information into the spreadsheet, and it will include values for the complete formula. At the point when you enter the number of servings, the spreadsheet will decide calories and nutrients per serving.

3). Ascertaining calories for full meals:

Regularly a supper comprises of a few distinct foods, some of which might be recipes that contain numerous ingredients. A model would be a pan-fried food (formula with numerous ingredients) with a side of rice (single ingredient). Calorie and supplement esteem for dinners can be calculated by entering the qualities for the individual ingredients and for the single-serving bit of recipes into a downloadable MS Excel® spreadsheet that is set up for this reason. Follow the means underneath to calculate the sustenance data for dinner.

1. Type the names of the ingredients and the recipes, alongside the measures of each into the spreadsheet. On the other hand, recipes might be replicated over from the Recipe Calculator above.

2. Look up the calories and nutrients for every individual ingredient in the right sum.

3. Enter the data into the Meal Calculator spreadsheet, including a number of servings for every individual ingredient or formula. The spreadsheet will, at that point, aggregate calories and nutrients giving you esteems for a solitary serving of the whole dinner.

Weight Index Calculator registers BMI record for grown-ups utilizing the following condition:

Weight Index Calculator Daily qualities depend on the 2000-calorie diet and 155 lbs. body weight (change). Real day-by-day supplement prerequisites may be diverse depending on your age, sexual orientation, level of physical action, restorative history, and different components.

THE BEST KETO CHAFFLE RECIPES TO TRY

Including recipes for some work of art, high-carb top picks that have been adjusted to be "fat bombs," which help keep your macros in balance, just as keep you from desiring every one of the things you, for the most part, cannot eat when you are attempting to get more fit.

A considerable amount of the in excess of 200 recipes require close to 10 to 15 minutes of planning time, and they taste as scrumptious and liberal as they sound–what about Chocolate Peanut Butter Pops, Mocha Cheesecake, or Almond Butter Bombs?

1. KETO CHAFFLE RECIPE

Keto Chaffle is the most recent new rage! The entire formula is just 3 net carbs all out.

INGREDIENTS

• 1 huge egg

• 1/2 c. Cheddar

• 2 tablespoons of almond flour

2. RICH and CREAMY CHAFFLES RECIPE

• 2 eggs

• 1 cup destroyed mozzarella

• 2 tablespoons almond flour

• 2 tablespoons cream cheddar

• 3/4 teaspoon preparing power

• 3 tablespoons water (discretionary)
• Makes 6 waffles.

3. ZUCCHINI CHUFFLES | ZUFFLES RECIPE

• 1 little zucchini, ground

• 1 egg

• 1 tablespoon parmesan

• Small bunch of destroyed mozzarella

• Basil and pepper to taste

• Mix all together and cook in a full-size waffle producer.

• Makes 2 full-size waffles and a meager raffle.

4. LIGHT and CRISPY CHAFFLES RECIPE

• 1 egg

• 1/3 cup cheddar

• 1/4 teaspoon heating powder

• 1/2 teaspoon ground flaxseed

• Shredded parmesan cheddar on top and base.

• Stir and cook in a mini waffle iron until fresh. – Kim H.

5. BACON CHEDDAR CHAFFLES RECIPE

• 1 egg

• 1.2 cup cheddar

• Bacon bits to taste

• Mix and cook until fresh.

6. BACON JALAPENO CHAFFLES RECIPE

• 1/2 cup destroyed Swiss/gruyere mix

• 1 egg

- 2 tablespoons cooked bacon pieces

- 1 tablespoon diced crisp jalapenos

- Cook until fresh. Works incredibly as a bun to a cheeseburger.

7. KETO CAULIFLOWER CHAFFLES RECIPE

You can make the most delightful keto cauliflower Chaffle formula with only a bunch of ingredients and a couple of moments! This formula will be your new top choice!

Ingredients

- 1 cup rice cauliflower

- 1/4 teaspoon Garlic Powder

- 1/4 teaspoon Ground Black Pepper

- 1/2 teaspoon Italian Seasoning

- 1/4 teaspoon salt

- 1/2 cup destroyed mozzarella cheddar or destroyed Mexican mix cheddar

- 1 Egg

- 1/2 cup destroyed parmesan cheddar

8. SANDWICH BREAD CHAFFLES RECIPE

- 1 egg

- 2 tablespoon almond flour

- 1 tablespoon mayo
- 1/8 teaspoon heating powder

- 1 teaspoon water

- Sweetener and garlic powder (discretionary)

- Makes 2 Chaffle, and you can undoubtedly slice them down the middle for a bun.

9. SWEET CHAFFLES RECIPES

To make Chaffle sweet, the conceivable outcomes are inestimable! You can just utilize the base formula and include some Keto-accommodating sugars.

In the event that you need to include some sweet seasoning after, you can sprinkle a wide range of Keto-accommodating magnificence on top. I like to utilize this Lecanto Maple Syrup. Something else, on the off chance that you need more than that, you can use the recipes beneath!

10. CHOCOLATE BROWNIE CHAFFLES

• Making the Keto Chocolate Brownies Batter.

• Stir and pour in the mini waffle producer.

• You can see the entire formula and a video here for how to make chocolate Chaffle

• Cook 5-7 minutes until firm. – Two Sleeve

11. MINT CHOCOLATE BROFFLE (BROWNIE WAFFLE)

• Use this keto brownie formula.

• Add hacked walnuts, and each broffle (brownie waffle) utilized 3 tablespoons of player for 7 min.

• The formula for the buttercream depends on Urvashi's maple walnut buttercream formula, just with mint rather than maple separate.

12. LEMON POUND CAKE CHAFFLES

Numerous individuals are cutting my lemon pound cake formula by 1/4 and making Cake Chaffle out of them.

Crusty fruit-filled treat CHAFFLES

• 1.2 cup mozzarella cheddar

• 1 egg

• Add the mozzarella to the waffle producer.

• Put the egg on top.

• Sprinkle on crusty fruit-filled treat zest and 5 sugar-free chocolate chips.

• Serve with margarine on top.

13. CREAM CHEESE CARROT CAKE CHAFFLES

• 2 tablespoons cream cheddar or a blend of 1-tablespoon cream cheddar and 2 tablespoons destroyed mozzarella cheddar

• 1/2 pat of margarine

• 1 tablespoon finely destroyed carrot

• 1 tablespoon of sugar of your decision. I utilized Splenda.

• 1 tablespoon almond flour

• 1 teaspoon pumpkin pie zest

• 1/2 teaspoon vanilla

• 1/2 teaspoon heating powder

• 1 egg

• OPTIONAL

I included 6 raisins, 1 tablespoon of destroyed coconut, and 1/2 tablespoon of pecans to the blender ingredients.

14. CREAM CHEESE FROSTING

• 1 tablespoon cream cheddar
• 1 pat spread

• 1 teaspoon sugar of decision. I utilized Cinnamon Brown Sugar without sugar syrup.

• Heat up, waffle creator. I utilized a mini Dash. I oiled with a silicon brush dunked in coconut oil.

• Microwave cream cheddar, mozzarella, and spread for 15 seconds to liquefy the cheeses to make consolidating simpler. I did this in an enchantment slug cup to mix.

- Add the remainder of the Chaffle ingredients to the blender cup and mix until smooth and consolidated.

- Add a player to a waffle creator. For the Dash, I included 2 stacking tablespoons, and it made 3 Chaffle.

- While making the Chaffle, heat up the spread and cream cheddar for the icing. Blend until smooth, and consolidate your sugar. Sprinkle over Chaffle as wanted.

15. CINNAMON CHAFFLES

- 1/2 cup mozzarella

- 1 egg

- 1 tbsp. vanilla concentrate

- 1/2 tsp preparing powder

- 1 tbsp. almond flour

- Sprinkle of cinnamon

- Mix together and cook until Chaffle are firm.

16. CINNAMON SWIRL CHAFFLES

- CHAFFLE:

- 1 oz. cream cheddar, mollified

- 1 huge egg, beaten

- 1 tsp vanilla concentrate

- 1 tbsp. almond flour, superfine

- 1 tbsp. Splenda

- 1 tsp cinnamon

- ICING:

- 1 oz. cream cheddar, mollified

- 1 tbsp. spread, unsalted

- 1 tbsp. Splenda

- 1/2 tsp vanilla

17. CINNAMON DRIZZLE:

- 1/2 tbsp. spread

- 1 tbsp. Splenda

- 1 tsp cinnamon

- Heat up waffle creator, and I brushed on coconut oil on my DASH. Stir up the Chaffle ingredients until smooth.
Utilize a spoon to include 2 piling tbsp. of the player to the waffle iron. It will make 3 little waffles. Cook to your ideal waffle freshness. I did 4 min. They resembled a delicate waffle.
Cool on a rack.

- Mix the icing and cinnamon shower in little dishes. Warmth in the microwave for 10 secs to find a workable pace consistency. Whirl on cooled waffles.

18. KETO SAUSAGE BALL

Portrayal

Keto Sausage Balls just contain four straightforward ingredients and make an extraordinary canapé or bite. They just contain 1 net carb and can without much of a stretch fit into your low carb or keto way of life.

INGREDIENTS

2 cups of almond flour

2 cups of cheddar

1 pound of pork wiener

8 oz. of cream cheddar

19. FAT HEAD PIZZA CRUST

INGREDIENTS

• 1 1/2 cups destroyed mozzarella

• 3/4 cup almond flour

• 2 tablespoons of cream cheddar, cubed

• 1 egg

• garlic powder, onion powder, and blended herbs for flavoring *see notes

20. Wild ox CHICKEN STUFFED AVOCADO

Portrayal

Wild ox Chicken Stuffed Avocado is a brisk formula utilizing stovetop bison chicken plunge and avocados. Making wild ox chicken plunge is extremely simple utilizing a stovetop too.

INGREDIENTS

• 2 5 oz. jars of chicken, depleted

• 2 tablespoons of whipped cream cheddar

• 2 tsp of dry Ranch flavoring blend

• ¼ cup of sans fat cheddar (utilize full fat with keto or low carb)

• 2 tablespoons of Frank's Buffalo Wing Sauce

• 1 medium avocado

21. ALMOND FLOUR BLUEBERRY PANCAKE Sakes

Depiction

Basic almond flour flapjacks made with just 6 ingredients. 2 net carbs per hotcake!

INGREDIENTS

2 huge eggs

⅓ Cup unsweetened almond milk 1-teaspoon vanilla concentrate
1 ¼-cup fine almond flour (utilized Bob's, Red Mill) ¼ teaspoon preparing pop
Touch of salt

Spread for lubing the skillet

22. BOSTON BROWN BREAD RECIPE

Ingredients

• 1 Egg

• 1 cup buttermilk or 1-cup milk with 1-tablespoon vinegar blended in

• 1/4 cup Molasses

• 1/4 cup Sugar

• 1 tablespoon Oil

• 1.5 cups Whole Wheat Flour

• 1/2 cup Cornmeal

• 2 teaspoons Baking Powder

• 1 teaspoon Ground Allspice

• 1/2 cup slashed pecans

• 1/4 cup Raisins

23. KETO CHEESE MUFFINS

Ingredients

• Vegetable oil for lubing the skillet

• 1 cup (112 g) Superfine Almond Flour

• 1/2 cup (85 g) Black Chia Seeds

• 2 teaspoons (2 teaspoons) Baking Powder

• 1/2 teaspoon (118.29 g) granulated garlic

- 4 enormous (4 huge) Eggs

- 1/4 cup (56.75 g) softened margarine

- 1/2 cup (56.5 g) ground cheddar

24. AIR FRYER BREADED CHICKEN WINGS

Ingredients

- 1 pound (453.59 g) chicken wings

- 3 tablespoons (3 tablespoons) Vegetable Oil

- 1/2 cup (62.5 g) All-Purpose Flour

- 1/2 teaspoon (0.5 teaspoon) Smoked Paprika

- 1/2 teaspoon (0.5 teaspoons) Garlic Powder

- 1/2 teaspoon (0.5 teaspoon) Salt

- 1/2 teaspoon (0.5 teaspoons) naturally squashed peppercorn

25. ONE STEP BRAZILIAN PAO DE QUEIJO BRAZILIAN CHEESE BREAD

Ingredients

- 1 cup (244 g) Whole Milk

- 1/2 cup (112 g) Oil

- 1 teaspoon (1 teaspoon) Salt

- 2 cups (240 g) Tapioca Flour

- 2 (2) Eggs

- 1.5 cups (150 g) destroyed parmesan cheddar

26. KETO ZUCCHINI WALNUT BREAD

Need to make a Keto Zucchini Bread, you will be super eager to eat and serve to other people? This formula with pecans is great!

Ingredients
• 1/2 cup (0.5 g) Trivia

• 3 (3) Eggs

• 1/2 cup (109 g) Ghee or Oil

• 1.5 cups (168 g) Superfine Almond Flour

• 1/2 cups (60 g) coconut flour

• 1 teaspoon (1 teaspoon) Baking Powder

• 1 teaspoon (1 teaspoon) Baking Soda

• 1/2 teaspoon (0.5 teaspoons) Ground Cinnamon

• 1/4 Teaspoon Ground Nutmeg

• 1/2 cup (250 g) Unsweetened Almond Milk

• 2 cups (248 g) destroyed zucchini

• 1 cup (117 g) cleaved pecans

27. KETO BREAD | NUT AND SEED BREAD

Ingredients

3 cups blended nuts and seeds left entire for instance

• 1/2 cup (61.5 g) pistachios

• 1/2 cup (71.5 g) almonds

• 1/2 cup (84 g) flaxseed

• 1/2 cup (58.5 g) pecans

• 1/2 cup (75 g) Sesame Seeds

• 1/2 cup (64.5 g) cashews Different ingredients

29

- 3 (3) Eggs

- 1/4 cup (56 ml) Oil

- 1/3 tsp (0.33 tsp) Salt

28. ONE STEP BRAZILIAN PAO DE QUEIJO BRAZILIAN CHEESE BREAD

Ingredients

- 1 cup (244 g) Whole Milk

- 1/2 cup (112 g) Oil

- 1 teaspoon (1 teaspoon) Salt

- 2 cups (240 g) Tapioca Flour

- 2 (2) Eggs

- 1.5 cups (150 g) destroyed parmesan cheddar

29. SWEET CREAM TRUFFLES

Ingredients

For the Truffle Center

- 2 cups (476 g) Heavy Whipping Cream

- 1/2 cup (91 g) powdered Swerve

For the Chocolate Coating

- 2 ounces (56.7 g) Sugar-Free Chocolate Chips

- 1 tablespoon (1 tablespoon) Butter

30. KETO MILKY BEARS| GUMMY BEAR RECIPE

These Keto Milky Bears are a fabulous sweet treat that will not take you out of ketosis. They are low carb, without gluten thus great you cannot simply eat one! Obviously superior to normal keto sticky bears.

Ingredients

• 1 13.5 ounces (1) Full-Fat Coconut Milk

• 2 bundles (2) unflavored gelatin, (3 tablespoons)

• 1/4 cup (62.5 g) Water

• 3 tablespoons (3 tablespoons) Trivia

• 2-3 drops (2) Panda Extract

31. KETO COCONUT PANNA COTTA

This straightforward Coconut Panna Cotta formula so sweet, smooth, and yummy that it will get one of your go-to pastries! In addition, it is low carb and dairy-free!

Ingredients

• 1/2 cup cold water

• 1 bundle unflavored gelatin, 1/4 oz. or 2.5 teaspoons

• 13.5 ounces Full-Fat Coconut Milk

• 1/8 cup Trivia

• 1 teaspoon unadulterated vanilla concentrate or coconut extricate

32. KETO CHOCOLATE CHEESECAKE BROWNIES

These Keto Chocolate Cheesecake Brownies are a chocolate cheesecake darlings dream! They are so acceptable you will not have the option to tell their low carb!

Ingredients

For the Brownie Batter

- 1/2 cup (90 g) Sugar-Free Chocolate Chips

- 1/2 cup (113.5 g) Butter

- 3 (3) Eggs

- 1/4 cup (0.25 g) Trivia, or other sugar

- 1 teaspoon (1 teaspoon) vanilla concentrate For the Cheesecake Batter
- 8 ounces (226.8 g) Cream Cheese, cubed and relaxed

- 1 (1) Egg

- 3 tablespoons (3 tablespoons) Trivia or other sugar

- 1 teaspoon (1 teaspoon) vanilla concentrate

33. KETO PIE CRUST

This 3-ingredient pat out Keto Pie Crust formula is a keto dieter's dream! No compelling reason to make crestless pies to keep it low carb. It is totally keto and vegan.

Ingredients

- 1 cup (112 g) Superfine Almond Flour

- 2 tablespoons (2 tablespoons) powdered Swerve
- 1/4 cup (54.5 g) Melted Coconut Oil

34. KETO MAPLE PECAN BLONDIES

These Keto Maple Pecan Blondies are the ideal sweet treat to fulfill your sweet tooth. They are wonderfully rich and shockingly low carb!
Ingredients
- 1 cup (112 g) Superfine Almond Flour

- 1/4 cup (30 g) coconut flour

- 2 teaspoons (2 teaspoons) Baking Powder

- 1/2 cup (91 g) Swerve

- 1/2 cup (113.5 g) Butter, softened

- 3 (3) Eggs

- 1 teaspoon (1 teaspoon) maple separate

- 3/4 cup (87.75 g) slashed pecans

35. KETO LASAGNA

Make this simple Keto Lasagna formula in your air fryer utilizing zucchini rather than conventional pasta noodles. It is so acceptable you will not miss the pasta!

Ingredients

- 1 cup marinara sauce

- 1 zucchini, cut into long, flimsy cuts For Meat Layer
- 1 cup finely slashed yellow onion

- 1 teaspoon Minced Garlic

- 1/2 pound-mass hot or mellow Italian frankfurter

- 1/2 cup ricotta cheddar

- 1/2 cup destroyed mozzarella cheddar

- 1/2 cup destroyed parmesan, isolated

- 1 Egg

- 1/2 teaspoon Garlic, minced

- 1/2 teaspoon Italian Seasoning

- 1/2 teaspoon Ground Black Pepper

36. KETO ALMOND PHIRNI KHEER

This Keto Almond Pharma Kheer is a heavenly Indian pastry formula that you are going to experience passionate feelings for! In addition, it is tasty; it is low carb as well!

Ingredients

- 3/4 cup (178.5 g) Heavy Whipping Cream

- 1 cup (250 g) Unsweetened Almond Milk

• 1/2 cup (56 g) Superfine Almond Flour

• 2 tablespoons (2 tablespoons) Trivia

• 1/2-1 teaspoon (0.5 teaspoons) Ground Cardamom

• 2-3 (2) Saffron Strands, squashed

37. TOMATO EGGPLANT SOUP

This is such an incredible vegan Tomato Eggplant Soup formula! Empty everything into your Instant Pot and you will have a bowl of great Mediterranean soup for supper in less than 30 minutes.

Ingredients
• 3 tablespoons Oil

• 2 tablespoons Minced Garlic

• 4 cups Eggplant, hacked

• 2 cups Tomatoes, hacked, or 1 14.5-ounce canned tomatoes, depleted

• 1 cup Onion, hacked

• 1 cup chimes pepper, cleaved

• 1/2 cup Water

• 1 teaspoon salt

• 1 teaspoon Ground Black Pepper

For Finishing

• 1/4 cup Basil, hacked

38. Hamburger KHEEMA MEATLOAF

Tired of normal meatloaf? Can't manage one more night of tacos to go through that ground hamburger? Make proper acquaintance with air fryer keto Indian Kheema meatloaf! Appreciate Indian food in a manner you may be comfortable with by making this Beef Kheema Meatloaf in your Air Fryer.

Ingredients

• 1 lb. Lean Ground Beef

• 2 Eggs

• 1 cup Onion, diced

• 1/4 cup Cilantro, hacked

• 1 tbsp. minced ginger

• 1 tbsp. Minced Garlic

• 2 tsp Gram Masala

• 1 tsp Salt

• 1 tsp Turmeric

• 1 tsp cayenne

• 1/2 tsp Ground Cinnamon

• 1/8 tsp Ground Cardamom

39. Weight COOKER LOW CARB WONTONS

Make these low carb wontons in your Instant pot, for the most delicate and succulent low carb wontons you have at any point had. Make these wontons without any wrappers, yet the entirety of the flavor of customary wontons.

Ingredients

• 1 pound (453.59 g) ground pork

• 1/4 cup (25 g) Green Onions, green and white parts blended

- 1/4 cup (4 g) Chopped Cilantro or Parsley

- 2 teaspoons (2 teaspoons) Soy Sauce

- 1 teaspoon (1 teaspoon) Oyster sauce

- 1 teaspoon (1 teaspoon) Ground Black Pepper

- ½ teaspoon (0.5 teaspoon) Salt

- 1 tablespoon (1 tablespoon) minced ginger

- 1 tablespoon (1 tablespoon) Minced Garlic

- 2 (2) Eggs

40. KETO CHICKEN BIRYANI

This Low Carb Chicken Biryani formula is Low-Carb Indian Food at its ideal. Cauliflower and ground chicken make up this fiery, heavenly low carb formula.

Ingredients

For Chicken

- 1 teaspoon Ghee

- 1 pound Ground Chicken

- 1 teaspoon salt

- 1/2 teaspoon Turmeric

- 1 teaspoon Gram Masala

- 1/2 teaspoon Ground Coriander

- 1/4 teaspoon Ground Cumin Vegetables
- 1 teaspoon Ghee

- 1 Red Onion, cut meager

- 1 Jalapeño pepper, diced

- 1 teaspoon ginger-garlic glue, (or 1/2 teaspoons minced garlic, 1/2 teaspoons minced ginger)

- 1/2 cup Water

- 1/2 cup Cilantro, slashed

- 1/4 cup mint leaves, slashed

- 2 cups cauliflower, riced

41. Moment POT CAULIFLOWER "Macintosh" AND CHEESE LOW CARB

Moment Pot Low Carb Keto Cauliflower and Cheese is a velvety, delightful side dish that you can make in your weight cooker for a definitive low carb comfort food!

Ingredients

- 2 cups (214 g) cauliflower, riced

- 2 tablespoon (2 tablespoons) Cream Cheese

- 1/2 cup (56.5 g) destroyed sharp cheddar

- 1/2 teaspoon (0.5 teaspoon) Salt

- 1/2 teaspoon (0.5 teaspoons) Ground Black Pepper

42. KETO HAM AND BEAN SOUP

No compelling reason to miss beans on a low carb diet. This Keto Ham and Bean Soup formula utilize a mystery, keto bean substitute that preferences simply like the genuine article.

Ingredients

- 1 cup (186 g) dried dark soybeans, doused to yield 2 cups beans

- 1 cup (160 g) onions, slashed

- 1 cup (101 g) slashed celery

- 4 cloves (4 cloves) Minced Garlic

- 1 teaspoon (1 teaspoon) Dried Oregano

- .5 to 1 teaspoon salt

- 1 teaspoon (1 teaspoon) Cajun Seasoning

- 1 teaspoon (1 teaspoon) Liquid Smoke

- 2 teaspoons (2 teaspoons) Tony Cheshire is universally handy flavoring

- 1 teaspoon (1 teaspoon) Louisiana Hot sauce

- 1 (1) substantial ham bone or 2 smoked ham sells

- 2 cups (280 g) slashed ham

- 2 cups (16.91 fly oz.) Water

43. Simple MANGO CARDAMOM PANNACOTTA

Low Carb Panna Cotta sets up rapidly and is a reviving summer dessert. Delicious, rich panna cotta joined with sweet mango. Ingredients
- 1 tablespoon (1 tablespoon) unflavored gelatin

- 2 cups (488 g) Fair life entire milk, (separated)

- 1 cup (165 g) mango

- 1 cup (238 g) Heavy Whipping Cream

- 1/2 cup (91 g) Swerve, or other sugar

- 1 teaspoon (1 teaspoon) Ground Cardamom

44. Smooth SHRIMP SCAMPI

Simple Low Carb Keto Creamy Shrimp Scampi from your moment pot or weight cooker, this one cooks quickly! Put it over some low carb noodles for a snappy supper.

Ingredients

- 2 tablespoons Butter

- 1 pound Shrimp, solidified

- 4 cloves Garlic, minced

- 1/4-1/2 teaspoons Red Pepper Flakes

- 1/2 teaspoons Smoked Paprika

- 2 cups Carbonado low carb pasta, (uncooked)

- 1 cup Chicken Broth

- 1/2 cup Half-and-Half

- 1/2 cup Parmesan Cheese

- Salt, to taste

- Ground Black Pepper, to taste

45. Moment POT SPAGHETTI SQUASH

When you make Spaghetti squash in the Instant pot, you will never make it another way. Eight minutes under tension, without cutting the squash, and you have the ideal low carb or veggie lover side dish.

Ingredients

- 1 Large Spaghetti Squash

- 1.5 cups Water, for the Instant Pot

46. TOMATO EGGPLANT SOUP

This is such an extraordinary vegan Tomato Eggplant Soup formula! Empty everything into your Instant Pot and you will have a magnificent Mediterranean soup for supper in less than 30 minutes.

Ingredients

- 3 tablespoons Oil

- 2 tablespoons Minced Garlic

- 4 cups Eggplant, slashed

- 2 cups Tomatoes, slashed, or 1 14.5 ounce canned tomatoes, depleted

- 1 cup Onion, slashed

- 1 cup ringer pepper, cleaved

- 1/2 cup Water

- 1 teaspoon salt

• 1 teaspoon Ground Black Pepper

47. Moment POT SAUERKRAUT SOUP RECIPE

Utilize your Instant Pot to make this flavorful, low-carb Sauerkraut Soup formula! It is a simple dump and cooks formula that cooks in a short time.
Ingredients

• 1 cup dried cannellini beans, drenched medium-term and depleted

• 14 oz. smoked frankfurters, cut down the middle longwise, and afterward cut into 1-inch pieces

• 1 cup sauerkraut with brackish water

• 3 Bay Leaves

• 1 cup onions, slashed

• 1 tablespoon Minced Garlic

• 1 teaspoon Salt

• 1 teaspoon Ground Black Pepper

• 4 cups Water

48. CHICKEN AND MUSHROOMS RECIPE

If you need to make a Chicken and Mushrooms Recipe, however, would prefer not to utilize canned soup, do I have only the thing for you! It is Keto and Instant Pot also!

Ingredients

• 2 tablespoons (2 tablespoons) Butter

• 1 cup (160 g) Sliced Onions

• 6 (6) Garlic Cloves, cut slender

• 1 cup (186 g) Mushrooms, cut into quarters

• 1 lb. (453.59 g) Boneless Skinless Chicken Thighs

• 4 cups (120 g) infant spinach

• 2 tablespoons (2 tablespoons) Water

• 1 teaspoonful of Dried Thyme or 3-4 sprigs crisp thyme

• 1 teaspoon (1 teaspoon) Salt

• 1 teaspoonful of Ground Black Pepper

• 1/2 cup (119 g) Heavy Whipping Cream

• 1 tablespoon (1 tablespoon) lemon juice

49. KETO SHRIMP SCAMPI

8 minutes from beginning to end to make this air fryer keto low carb shrimp scampi. So easy to make, so heavenly, you will have a hard time believing it. Ingredients
• 4 tablespoons (4 tablespoons) Butter

• 1 tablespoon (1 tablespoon) lemon juice

• 1 tablespoon (1 tablespoon) Minced Garlic

• 2 teaspoons (2 teaspoons) Red Pepper Flakes

• 1 tablespoon (1 tablespoon) hacked chives, or 1 teaspoon dried chives

• 1 tablespoon (1 tablespoon) hacked crisp basil, or 1 teaspoon dried basil

• 2 tablespoons of Chicken Stock, (or white wine)

• 1 lb. (453.59 g) defrosted shrimp, (21-25 check)

50. Essential INDIAN CURRY RECIPE | PRESSURE COOKER CURRY RECIPE

This Basic Indian Curry is a tasty customary Indian curry formula made in the Instant Pot! This curry formula is low-carb and stuffed with Indian flavor. Ingredients
• 1 pound (453.59 g) Boneless Pork Shoulder, diced into 2 inch 3D squares

• 1.5 cups (240 g) onions, hacked

• 1 cup (242 g) Canned Tomatoes, undrained

• 1 tablespoon (1 tablespoon) Minced Garlic

- 1 tablespoon minced ginger

- 2 teaspoons (2 teaspoons) Garam Masala, separated

- 1 teaspoon (1 teaspoon) Salt

- 1 teaspoon (1 teaspoon) Turmeric

- 1/4-1 teaspoon (0.25 teaspoon) Cayenne

- 2 tablespoons (2 tablespoons) Water

51. CHICKEN TIKKA MASALA

Make simple, real Chicken Tikka Masala comfortable in your Instant Pot or weight cooker! It is by a wide margin the simplest method to make Chicken Tikka Masala.

Ingredients

Marinate the chicken

- 1 ½ pound (680.39 g) Boneless Skinless Chicken Thighs, (bosom or thighs), cut into enormous pieces

- ½ cups (100 g) Greek Yogurt

- 4 cloves (4 cloves) Garlic, minced

- 2 teaspoons (2 teaspoons) minced ginger, minced

- ½ teaspoon (0.5 teaspoon) Turmeric

- ¼ teaspoon (0.25 teaspoon) Cayenne

- ½ teaspoon (0.5 teaspoons) Smoked Paprika, for shading and a somewhat smoky taste

- 1 teaspoon (1 teaspoon) Salt

- 1 teaspoon (1 teaspoon) Garam Masala

- 1/2 teaspoon (0.5 teaspoons) Ground Cumin

- 1 teaspoon (1 teaspoon) Liquid Smoke, (overlook if inaccessible)

52. Simple TRADITIONAL KETO CHAFFLE

INGREDIENTS

• 1 Egg

• 1/2 cup Shredded Cheddar Cheese Directions
1. Preheat mini waffle creator.

2. In a cup, whisk the egg until beaten.

3. Add destroyed cheddar and mix to consolidate.

4. When the waffle creator is warmed, cautiously pour 1/2 of the hitter in the waffle producer and close the top. Permit to cook for 3-5 minutes.

5. Carefully expel from the waffle producer and put in a safe spot for 2-3 minutes to fresh up.

6. Repeat guidelines again for the second Chaffle.

53. KETO STRAWBERRY SHORTCAKE CHAFFLE

INGREDIENTS

• 1 Egg

• 1 tbsp. Heavy Whipping Cream

• 1 tsp Coconut Flour

• 2 tbsp. Lakanto Golden Sweetener (Use butter together for 20% off)

• 1/2 tsp Cake Batter Extract

• 1/4 tsp Baking powder

54. KETO PUMPKIN CHEESECAKE CHAFFLE

INGREDIENTS

PUMPKIN CHAFFLE

• 1 Egg
• 1/2 cup Mozzarella Cheese

- 1 1/2 tbsp. Pumpkin Puree (100% pumpkin)

- 1 tbsp. Almond Flour

- 1 tbsp. Lakanto Golden Sweetener, or decision of sugar

- 2 tsp Heavy Cream

- 1 tsp Cream Cheese, relaxed

- 1/2 tsp Pumpkin Spice

- 1/2 tsp Baking Powder

- 1/2 tsp Vanilla

- 1 tsp Choc zero Maple Syrup or 1/8 tsp Maple Extract

55. Tasty KETO PIZZA CHAFFLE RECIPE

INGREDIENTS

CHAFFLE CRUST

- 1 Egg

- 1/2 cup Mozzarella Cheese

- 1 tsp Coconut Flour

- 1/4 tsp Baking Powder

- 1/8 tsp Garlic Powder

- 1/8 tsp Italian Seasoning

- Pinch of Salt

56. PIZZA TOPPING

- 1 tbsp. Rao's Marinara Sauce

- 1/2 cup Mozzarella Cheese

- 3 Pepperoni's, cut into four

- Shredded Parmesan Cheese, discretionary

• Parsley, discretionary

57. BEST OREO KETO CHAFFLES

INGREDIENTS

CHOCOLATE CHAFFLE

• 1 Egg

• 1 1/2 tbsp. Unsweetened Cocoa

• 2 tbsp. Lakanto Monk fruit or decision of sugar

• 1 tbsp. Heavy Cream

• 1 tsp Coconut Flour

• 1/2 tsp Baking Powder

• 1/2 tsp Vanilla

• Whipped Cream (interchange icing formula in notes beneath) Guidelines
1. Preheat mini waffle producer.

2. In a small bowl, join all Chaffle ingredients.

3. Pour a portion of the Chaffle blend into the focal point of the waffle iron. Permit to cook for 3-5 minutes.

58. KETO PEANUT BUTTER CUP CHAFFLE

INGREDIENTS
CHAFFLE

• 1 Egg

• 1 tbsp. Heavy Cream

• 1 tbsp. Unsweetened Cocoa

• 1 tbsp. Lakanto Powdered Sweetener

• 1 tsp Coconut Flour

• 1/2 tsp Vanilla Extract

- 1/2 Cake Batter Flavor (we utilize this)

- 1/4 tsp Baking Powder

- 3 tbsp. All regular Peanut Butter

- 2 tsp Lakanto Powdered Sweetener

- 2 tbsp. Heavy Cream

59. KETO SNICKERDOODLE CHAFFLE

INGREDIENTS

- 1 Egg

- 1/2 cup Mozzarella Cheese

- 2 tbsp. Almond Flour

- 1 tbsp. Lakanto Golden Sweetener

- 1/2 tsp Vanilla Extract

- 1/4 tsp Cinnamon

- 1/2 tsp Baking Powder

- 1/4 tsp Cream of tartar, discretionary Covering
- 1 tbsp. Butter

- 2 tbsp. Lakanto Classic Sweetener

- 1/2 tsp Cinnamon

1. Preheat your mini waffle producer.

2. In a little bowl, join all Chaffle ingredients.

3. Pour a portion of the Chaffle blend on to the focal point of the waffle iron. Permit to cook for 3-5 minutes.

4. Carefully expel and rehash for the second Chaffle. Permit Chaffle to cool so they fresh.

5. In a little bowl, consolidate sugar and cinnamon for covering.

6. Melt spread in a little microwave-safe bowl and brush the Chaffle with the margarine.

7. Sprinkle sugar and cinnamon blend on the two sides of the Chaffle once they are brushed with margarine.

60. WHITE BREAD KETO CHAFFLE | WONDER BREAD CHAFFLE

INGREDIENTS

• 1 Egg

• 3 tbsp. Almond Flour

• 1 tbsp. Mayonnaise

• 1/4 tsp Baking Powder

• 1 tsp Water Guidelines
1. Preheat mini waffle producer.

2. In a cup, whisk the egg until beaten.
3. Add almond flour, mayonnaise, heating powder, and water.

4. When the waffle producer is warmed, cautiously pour 1/2 of the hitter in the waffle creator and close the top. Permit to cook for 3-5 minutes.

5. Carefully expel from the waffle creator and put in a safe spot for 2-3 minutes to fresh up.

6. Repeat directions again for the second Chaffle.

61. BEST OREO KETO CHAFFLES

INGREDIENTS

CHOCOLATE CHAFFLE

• 1 Egg

• 1 1/2 tbsp. Unsweetened Cocoa

• 2 tbsp. Lakanto Monk fruit or decision of sugar

• 1 tbsp. Heavy Cream

• 1 tsp Coconut Flour

• 1/2 tsp Baking Powder

• 1/2 tsp Vanilla

• Whipped Cream (exchange icing formula in notes beneath) Guidelines
1. Preheat mini waffle producer.

2. In a small bowl, join all Chaffle ingredients.

3. Pour a portion of the Chaffle blend into the focal point of the waffle iron. Permit to cook for 3-5 minutes.

62. KETO CHOCOLATE CHIP CHAFFLE KETO RECIPE

Ingredients

• 1 egg

• 1 tbsp. substantial whipping cream

• 1/2 tsp coconut flour

• 1 3/4 tsp Lakanto monk fruit brilliant can utilize pretty much to change the sweetness

• 1/4 tsp preparing powder

• Pinch of salt

• 1 tbsp. Lily's Chocolate Chips

1. Turn on the waffle creator with the goal that it warms up.

2. In a little bowl, join all ingredients with the exception of the chocolate chips and mix well until consolidated.

3. Grease waffle producer, at that point, pour half of the hitter onto the base plate of the waffle creator.

4. Cook it for 5 minutes or until the chocolate chip Chaffle pastry is brilliant dark colored at that point expel from waffle creator with a fork, being mindful so as not to burn your fingers.

63. KETO STRAWBERRY CHEESECAKE SHAKE

INGREDIENTS

• 1 cup Almond Milk, unsweetened

• 2oz Cream cheddar
• 1/2 cup Strawberries

• 2 tbsp. Heavy cream

• 1 tbsp. Lakanto monk fruit or decision of sugar

• 1/2 tsp Vanilla

• 1 tbsp. Choc Zero Strawberry Syrup, discretionary Directions
1. Add every one of the ingredients into a blender and mix until smooth. Include ice-blocks varying. Appreciate!

64. KETO TACO CHAFFLE RECIPE (CRISPY TACO SHELLS)

Ingredients

• 1 egg white

• 1/4 cup Monterey jack cheddar, destroyed (stuffed firmly)

• 1/4-cup sharp cheddar, destroyed (stuffed firmly)

• 3/4 tsp water

• 1 tsp coconut flour

• 1/4 tsp preparing powder

• 1/8 tsp stew powder

• Pinch of salt

1. Plug the Dash Mini Waffle Maker in the divider and oil delicately once it is hot.

2. Combine the entirety of the ingredients in a bowl and mix to consolidate.

3. Spoon out 1/2 of the player on the waffle creator and close top. Set a clock for 4 minutes and do not lift the cover until the cooking time is finished. In the event that you do, it will resemble the taco Chaffle shell is not set up appropriately. However, it will. You need to let it cook the whole 4 minutes before lifting the cover.

65. MAPLE PUMPKIN KETO WAFFLE RECIPE (CHAFFLE)

Ingredients

• 2 eggs

• 3/4 tsp heating powder

• 2 tsp pumpkin puree (100% pumpkin)

• 3/4 tsp pumpkin pie zest

• 4 tsp substantial whipping cream

• 2 tsp Lakanto Sugar-Free Maple Syrup

• 1 tsp coconut flour

• 1/2 cup mozzarella cheddar, destroyed

• 1/2 tsp vanilla

• Pinch of salt

1. Turn on a waffle or Chaffle producer. I utilize the Dash Mini Waffle Maker.

2. In a little bowl, join all ingredients.

3. Cover the scramble mini waffle producer with 1/4 of the player and cook for 3-4 minutes.

4. Repeat 3 additional occasions until you have made 4 Maple Syrup Pumpkin Keto Waffles (Chaffle).

5. Serve with without sugar maple syrup or keto frozen yogurt.

66. KETO CHAFFLE BREAKFAST SANDWICH

Ingredients

• 1 egg

• 1/2 cup Monterey Jack Cheese

• 1 tablespoon almond flour

• 2 tablespoons spread Directions
1. In a little bowl, blend the egg, almond flour, and Monterey Jack Cheese.

2. Pour a portion of the hitter into your mini waffle creator and cook for 3-4 minutes. At that point, cook the remainder of the player to make a second Chaffle.

3. In a little container, dissolve 2 tablespoons of spread. Include the Chaffle and cook each side for 2 minutes. Pushing down while they are cooking gently on the highest point of them, so they are fresh up better.

4. Remove from the container and let sit for 2 minutes.

67. MINI KETO PIZZA RECIPE

Ingredients

• 1/2 cup Shredded Mozzarella cheddar

• 1 tablespoon almond flour

• 1/2 tsp heating powder

• 1 egg

• 1/4 tsp garlic powder

• 1/4 tsp basil

• 2 tablespoons low carb pasta sauce

• 2 tablespoons mozzarella cheddar Guidelines
1. While the waffle producer is warming up, in a bowl blend mozzarella cheddar, preparing powder, garlic, premise, egg, and almond flour.

2. Pour 1/2 the blend into your mini waffle producer.

3. Cook it for 3-5 min. until your pizza waffle is totally cooked. On the off chance that you check it and the waffle adheres to the waffle creator, let it cook for one more moment or two.

68. SUGAR-FREE VANILLA BUTTERCREAM FROSTING

Ingredients

• 1 cup margarine room temperature

• 1.5 cups swerve confectioner

• 2 tbsp. Heavy Whipping Cream

• 1 tsp vanilla concentrate Guidelines
1. Place your margarine and swerve in the bowl of your blender. Combine them on low speed until the sugar is joined.

2. Mix in the substantial cream and the vanilla concentrate.

3. Turn the blender up to medium-fast and keep blending for 6-8 minutes until light and feathery.

69. KETO BLUEBERRY CHAFFLE

A scrumptious keto blueberry waffles are, in fact, called a Keto Chaffle! What's more, a kid is it delish! Consummately sweet, with succulent blueberries,
these blueberry keto Chaffle taste extraordinary and are low carb and keto well disposed.

Ingredients

• 1 cup of mozzarella cheddar

• 2 tablespoons almond flour

• 1 tsp preparing powder

• 2 eggs

• 1 tsp cinnamon

• 2 tsp of Swerve

•3 tablespoon blueberries Directions
1. Heat up your Dash mini waffle creator.

2. In a blending bowl include the mozzarella cheddar, almond flour, preparing powder, eggs, cinnamon, swerve, and blueberries. Blend well, so every one of the ingredients is combined.

3. Spray your mini waffle creator with non-stick cooking splash.

4. Add shortly less than 1/4 a cup of blueberry keto waffle hitter.

70. GREEK MARINATED FETA AND OLIVES

Ingredients

• 1 cup olive oil

• 1/4 teaspoon oregano

• 1/4 teaspoon thyme

• 1/2 teaspoon dried rosemary

• 1 cup kalamata olives

• 1 cup of green olives

• 1/2 pound feta

1. In a little pot heat, the oil, oregano, thyme, rosemary together over medium warmth for 5 minutes to imbue the oil with the herbs.

2. Set the oil to the side and enable it to cool for 15 minutes.

3. Cut the feta into 1/2 inch 3D shapes.

71. AIR FRYER PEANUT CHICKEN

Not many things state "Thai food" like Peanut Chicken. This Peanut Chicken formula takes the dish to an unheard-of level and is effectively made in your air fryer!

Ingredients

• 1 pound Bone-in Skin-on Chicken Thighs For the Sauce
• 1/4 cup Creamy Peanut Butter

• 1 tablespoon Sriracha Sauce, (modify for your zest needs)

• 1 tablespoon Soy Sauce

• 2 tablespoons sweet chili sauce

• 2 tablespoons limejuice

• 1 teaspoon Minced Garlic

• 1 teaspoon minced ginger

• 1/2 teaspoon salt, to taste

• 1/2 cup high temporary water

72. GREEN BEANS WITH BACON

Right now, Pot Green Beans with Bacon formula is a fast, low carb, and nutritious dish that can be eaten either as a side dish or as a low carb dinner. Just beans, bacon, and a couple of seasonings make this a quick and simple dish.
Ingredients

• 1 cup (160 g) onion, diced

• 5 cuts (5 cuts) Bacon, diced

• 6 cups (660 g) green beans cut in

73. KETO BUFFALO CHICKEN CASSEROLE

This Buffalo Chicken Casserole is as flavorful filling dish with the perfect measure of kick! The ideal weeknight supper requires little exertion to make. Ingredients
• 4 cups rotisserie chicken, destroyed

• 1/2 cup Onion, slashed

• 1/4 cup Cream

• 1/4 cup hot wing sauce

• 1/4 cup blue cheddar, disintegrated

• 2 ounces Cream Cheese, diced

- Pepper

- 1/4 cup Green Onions, slashed

74. GERMAN RED CABBAGE

Appreciate this customary German Red Cabbage formula made in a non-conventional way! Make this wonderfully prepared side dish directly in your Instant Pot!

Ingredients

- 6 cups red cabbage, cleaved

- 3 Granny Smith Apples, little, cut 1 inch thick

- 2 tablespoons liquefied margarine or oil

- 1/3 cup Apple Cider Vinegar

- 2-3 tablespoons Sugar

- 1 teaspoon salt

- 1/2 teaspoon Ground Black Pepper

- 1/4 teaspoon Ground Cloves

- 2 sound leaves

75. MAPLE PECAN BARS WITH SEA SALT

Ingredients

For the Crust

- Non-Stick Spray

- 1/3 cup Butter, mellowed

- 1/4 cup Brown Sugar, immovably stuffed

- 1 cup All-Purpose Flour

- 1/4 kosher tea Salt

- 4 TBS Butter (1/2 stick), diced

- 1/2 cup Brown Sugar

- 1/4 cup Pure Maple Syrup

- 1/4 cup Whole Milk

- 1/4 tea Vanilla concentrate

76. Moment POT VEGETARIAN CHILI

Ingredients
- 1 cup Onion, cleaved

- 1 cup Canned Fire Roasted Tomatoes

- 1.5 tablespoons Minced Garlic

- 3 corn tortillas

- 1 tablespoon Chipotle Chile in Adobo Sauce, cleaved

- 1 tablespoon Mexican Red Chili Powder, (not cayenne)

- 2 teaspoons Ground Cumin

- 2 teaspoons salt

- 1 teaspoon Dried Oregano

- 1 cup Water

- 1/2 cup dried pinto beans, doused medium-term or for 1 hour in heated water

- 1/2 cup dried dark beans, splashed medium-term or for 1 hour in high temp water

- 2 cups corn, new or defrosted solidified corn

- 2 cups zucchini, hacked

77. KETO ALMENDRADOS COOKIES | SPANISH ALMOND KETO COOKIES

Ingredients

• 1.5 cups Superfine Almond Flour

• 1/2 cup Swerve

• 1 huge Egg

• 1 teaspoon Lemon Extract

• 1 tablespoon lemon get-up-and-go

• 24 whitened almonds

1. In a medium bowl, beat egg. Include almond flour, swerve and lemon and combine to make a strong mixture. Cover and refrigerate for 1-2 hours.

2. Preheat stove to 350 degrees. Line a heating sheet with material paper.

3. pinching off bits of batter about the size of a pecan, fold them into balls.

78. KETO TACO

Prep. Time: 11 minutes/Cook time: 20 minutes/Serves 3

Need to begin the day surprising? Morning keto is such an astounding beginning to a delightful day. Light and superb with a lot of splendid hues and feelings.

8 oz. Mozzarella cheddar, destroyed; 6 Eggs, enormous 2 tbsp. Margarine

3 Bacon stripes ½ Avocado 1 oz. Cheddar, destroyed Pepper and salt to taste

79. KETO OMELET WITH GOAT CHEESE AND SPINACH

Prep. Time: 5 minutes

3 Large eggs 1 Medium green onion 1 oz. Goat cheddar ¼ Onion

2 tbsp. Margarine 2 cups Spinach 2 tbsp. Substantial cream Salt and pepper to taste

80. CHICKEN AND CHEESE QUESADILLA

Prep. Time: 10 minutes/Serves 4

For capsules: 6 Eggs 4 oz. Coconut flour 6 oz. Substantial cream ½ tsp. Thickener Pink salt and pepper 1 tbsp. Olive oil for fricasseeing

For the quesadilla: 4 oz. Cheddar destroyed 8 oz. Chicken bosom cooked and destroyed 1 tbsp. Parsley, cleaved (discretionary)

81. Veggie lover SCRAMBLE

Prep. Time: 5 minutes/Serves 5

The formula is anything to get ready; however, delectable avocados, tomatoes, and cheeses will lift your spirits and empower for extraordinary deeds. 1 lb. Tofu cheddar 3 tbsp. Avocado oil 2 tbsp. Cleaved onion 1½ tbsp. Food yeast ½ tsp. Garlic powder
½ tsp. Turmeric ½ tsp. Salt 1-cup Spinach 3 Grape tomatoes 3 oz. Vegan Cheddar Cheese

82. BURGER WITH GUACAMOLE AND EGG

At times toward the beginning of the day, you truly need a succulent burger with different flavors. Along these lines, I have arranged for you this magnificent formula. Delicious meat, lively guacamole, an egg, and 10 minutes are all you have to make the most of your most loved keto burgher. Everybody around will need the equivalent.

5 oz. Ground hamburger 4 Bacon, cuts 3 oz. Guacamole 1 Egg

1 tbsp. Olive oil (for singing) ½ tsp. Italian flavoring Salt and pepper to taste

83. STUFFED AVOCADO

1 Avocado hollowed and cut down the middle 1 tbsp. Margarine salted 3 large eggs.

3 cuts of bacon cut into little pieces Salt and dark pepper, to taste

84. OMELET WITH MUSHROOMS AND GOAT CHEESE

Prep. Time: 6 minutes/Serves 1

3 Large eggs 2 tsp. overwhelming cream 3 oz. Cleaved mushrooms 1 tsp. Olive oil

2 oz. Disintegrated goat cheddar seasoning to taste Green onions for decorating

85. FAT BOMBS

Neapolitan Fatty Bombs

Prep. Time: 10 minutes/Serves 24

½ cup Butter ½ cup Coconut oil ½ cup Sour cream ½ cup Cream cheddar 2 tbsp. Erythritol

25 drops Liquid stevia 2 tbsp. Cocoa powder 1 tsp. Vanilla concentrate 2 medium strawberries

86. CHOCOLATE-COCONUT FAT BOMBS WITH ALMONDS

Prep. Time: 5 minutes/Serves 12

1 cup Coconut chips 3 tbsp. Fat coconut milk 3 tbsp. Coconut oil (softened) ½ tsp. Vanilla concentrate

4 oz. Chocolate chips, no sugar a spot of salt 2 oz. Keto-accommodating sugar 24 Almond, pieces

87. Fiery FAT BOMBS

Prep. Time: 6 minutes/Serves 12

6 MCT powder scoops 10 Liquid stevia's, drops 1 tsp. Turmeric 1 tbsp. Dark sesame seeds Squeeze Chinese 5 Spice Blend a spot of dark pepper ½ tsp. Cinnamon 2½ fl. oz. Warm water

88. Espresso FAT BOMBS

Prep. Time: 5 minutes/Serves 12

4 oz. Margarine 2 oz. Ghee spread (dissolved) 2 oz. overwhelming cream 1 tbsp. Milk to your taste Double coffee

2 oz. Keto-accommodating sugar of your decision 1 tsp. Vanilla concentrate a spot of salt

89. ALMOND COCONUT FAT BOMBS

Prep. Time: 5 minutes/Serves 10

2 fl. oz. Almond oil 2 fl. oz. Coconut oil

2 tbsp. Cocoa powder 2 fl. oz. Erythritol, to your taste

90. PUMPKIN FAT SPICE BOMBS

Time: 5 minutes/Serves 9

8 oz. crude cashews 4 oz. crude macadamia nuts 4 oz. Coconut chips 3 fl. oz. Pumpkin puree

2 tbsp. MCT oils 2 tsp. Cinnamon, ground 2 tsp. Ginger, and ground Neutral oil (avocado oil)

91. Cheddar FAT BOMBS IN BACON

Time: 5 minutes

Serves 20
8 oz. Mozzarella cheddar 4 tbsp. Almond flour 4 tbsp. Spread, softened 3 tbsp. Psyllium powder 1 Egg Salt, to taste 1 tsp. Dark pepper 1/8 tsp. Garlic powder 1/8 tsp. Onion powder 20 Bacon, cuts 1-cup oil or fat (for singing) Plates of mixed greens

Vegetable Salad with Bacon and Cheese

Cook time: 10 minutes, Serves 6

4 oz. Lettuce 3 oz. Spinach 2 oz. Wavy cabbage 6 cuts of cooked bacon 12 pcs. Grape tomato

92. A plate of mixed greens WITH CHICKEN BREAST AND GREENS

Time: 10 minutes/ Serves 2

2 tbsp. Pesto sauce 2 fl. oz. Balsamic vinegar 1 tsp. Olive oil 6 oz. Chicken bosom 4-cup spring greens

1 oz. New mozzarella ¼ Avocado, diced 6 Cherry tomatoes 1 tbsp. Crisp basil for beautification

93. SALMON SALAD

Time: 5 minutes

2 Sheets of lettuce 6 leaves, Fresh basil, finely hacked ½ tsp. Garlic powder 1 tsp. Lemon juice

4 tbsp. Mayonnaise 5 oz. Salmon 1 oz. Red onion, hacked ½ Avocado, diced 2 tbsp. Parmesan cheddar, diced

94. Straightforward CABBAGE AND EGG KETO SALAD

Time: 10 minutes

1 lb. Cauliflower blossoms 4 oz. Keto mayonnaise 1 tsp. Yellow mustard 1½ tsp. New dill Ground dark pepper and salt, to taste 2 oz. finely hacked dill

1 Celery stalk, finely hacked 2 oz. Red onion hacked 1 tbsp. Salted keto cucumber, slashed 6 Hard-bubbled eggs, hacked Paprika, for embellish

95. LIGHT PEA AND GREEN ONION SALAD

Cook time: 10 minutes/Serves

2 oz. Pea 2 tsp. Green onions ½ tsp. Soy sauce 2 tsp. Olive oil

½ tsp. Apple vinegar ½ tsp. Sesame oil ½ tsp. Sesame seeds Garlic powder, to taste.

96. KETO-SALSA WITH AVOCADO AND SHRIMPS

Prep. Time: 10 minutes

8 oz. Stripped crude shrimp 1 tbsp. Olive oil 1 Lemon (juice) 1 Avocado, diced 1 Tomato, diced

1 Cucumber, diced 1/4 Onion, diced 2 oz. Cilantro, cleaved Salt and dark pepper, to taste.

97. KETO SALAD TACO

1 lb. Ground hamburger from grass-encouraged meat 1 tsp. Ground cumin ½ tsp. Bean stew powder 1 tbsp. Garlic powder ½ tbsp. Paprika Salt and pepper, a 5 cups Roman lettuce

1 Tomato 4 oz. Cheddar 4 oz. Cilantro 1 Avocado 4 oz. Most loved salsa 2 little limes 1 cup Cucumber, cut Tidbits

98. Snappy Keto Bread

Prep. Time: 5 minutes/Cook time: 10 minutes/Serves 10

2 tbsp. Almond flour ½ tbsp. Coconut flour 1/4 tsp. Heating powder 1 Egg

½ tbsp. Ghee or margarine 1 tbsp. Unsweetened milk of your choice

99. Vitality KETO BARS WITH NUTS AND SEEDS

Prep. Time: 10 minutes

Serves 8

2 tbsp. Margarine or coconut oil 2 fl. oz. Sans sugar 1 tsp. Vanilla concentrate 8 oz. Almond, slashed 8 oz. Crude macadamia nuts (finely cleaved) 4 oz. Pumpkin seed

2 tbsp. Hemp seed 1-2 tsp. Keto sugar (if important) 4 oz. Low sugar chocolate chips ½ tsp. Coconut or margarine, or ghee oil

100. LOW-CARB FLAX BREAD

Time: 10 minutes - Cook time: 15 minutes - Serves 8
1 oz. Almond flour 1½ Flaxseed 1 tsp. Heating powder Salt, to taste ½ tsp. Vinegar

4 drops liquid stevia 3 oz. Crude whisked egg 1 fl. oz. — coconut oil or margarine (softened).

101. Keto Mini Pizza

Time: 5 minutes - Cook time: 15 minutes - Serves 4

1 oz. Keto mayonnaise 1 tbsp. raw eggs 2 tsp. Coconut oil melted 2 tsp. Almond flour
1 tsp. Coconut flour ½ tsp. Psyllium powder a pinch of baking powder and baking soda

102. Baked Eggs with Ham and Asparagus

Time: 5 minutes - Cook time: 15 minutes - Serves

6 Eggs 6 slices (about 4 oz.) Italian ham 8 oz. Asparagus
A few sprigs of fresh marjoram 1 tbsp. Butter or ghee

103. Eggplant Keto Chips

Time: 5 minutes - Cook time: 20 minutes - Serves 4

2 fl. oz. Olive oil 1 large eggplant (thinly sliced) Salt and pepper to taste 1 tsp. Garlic powder ½ tsp. Dry basil ½ tsp. Dried oregano 2 tbsp. Parmesan cheese

104. Cheese Keto Sticks

Time: 5 minutes - Cook time: 20 minutes - Serves 3

3 Mozzarella cheese sticks (cut in half) 4 oz. Almond flour 1 tbsp. Italian seasoning mixes 2 tbsp. Grated parmesan cheese

105. Chicken Keto Nuggets

Time: 15 minutes - Cook time: 5 hours - Serves 4

1 oz. Whipped egg whites 1 oz. Chicken breast cooked and minced ½ oz. Coconut flour ½ tsp. Baking powder
1 fl. oz. Olive oil ½ oz.
Softened margarine 1 oz. Fatty 40% cream Salt, pepper, a spot of garlic powder, discretionary

1. Blend destroyed chicken in with coconut flour, heating powder, and flavoring. The blend should look extremely dry.

2. Include spread and blend once more. Include whipped egg whites and blend until smooth.

3. Empty olive oil into a little non-stick container. Spread the chicken-egg blend in little pieces and fry for around 1 moment on each side.

4. Present with whipped cream, weakened with water, similar to "milk."

Calories: 136. Fat: 41 g. Protein: 9 g. Carbs: 2

106. Champignon Keto Burger

Time: 5 minutes / Serves 4

3 Large champignons. Olive oil 2 tbsps. Balsamic vinegar 3 slices of bacon 4 oz. Ground meat ½ tsp. Garlic powder
½ tsp. Onion powder ½ tsp. Worcestershire Sauce 1 cheddar, cut 1 Slice of tomato 2 oz. Blended greens or arugula 1 tbsp. Low-sugar ketchup

107. Nourishing Beef Soup

Time: 10 minutes / Serves

1 lb. Ground beef 5 slices of bacon 1 tbsp. Olive oil 1 tbsp. 1½-cup Bone broth
1-cup Shredded cheddar 2 fl. oz. Fat whipped cream 2 tsp. Psyllium powder 4 oz. Shredded cheddar cheese ½ oz. Chopped green onions ½-cup Sour cream

108. Keto Cheeseburger with Bacon

Time: 10 minutes, Serves 2

For the dough: 8 oz. Mozzarella, shredded 4 oz. Almond flour 1 tbsp. Cream cheese
For the filling: 6oz. Ground beef 2 slice of cheddar cheese, cut into quarters

107. Spicy Keto Soup with Mushrooms

Time: 10 minutes, Serves 4

1 tbsp. Olive oil 1 onion (thinly sliced) 1 tbsp. Fresh grated ginger 3 Garlic, cloves (finely chopped) 1 tsp. Chile 1 tbsp. Fish sauce
2 fl. oz. Soy sauce 2 fl. oz. Rice vinegar 4 oz. Mushrooms (thinly sliced) 4 Hard-boiled eggs 2-3 packets of shirataki noodles 5 cup Bone broth

108. Greek Keto Moussaka

Time: 10 minutes

Serves 3
For the filling: ½ Chopped eggplant 10 oz. Minced chicken 3 tbsp. Marinara sauce 1 Minced garlic ½ Chopped onion 1 tsp. Dried oregano 1 tsp. Paprika

½ tsp. Ground cinnamon 2 tbsp. Olive oil

For the sauce: 3 tbsp. Liberal cream 3 tbsp. Cream cheddar 3 oz. Squashed cheddar 1 Minced garlic

109. Almond Pancakes with Shrimp and Cheese

Time: 10 minutes/Serves 8

1 lb. Shrimp cooked and slashed 2 oz. Almond flour 1 Whisked egg 2 oz. Mozzarella, destroyed

3 tbsp. Parmesan cheddar, ground 1 tbsp. Crisp dill, slashed 1½ tbsp. Olive or coconut oil, for broiling Salt and pepper, to taste.

110. Baked Halibut Cheese Breaded

Time: 10 minutes, Serves 6

2 lb. Halibut (about 6 fillets) 1 tbsp. Butter 3 tbsp. Grated parmesan cheese 1 tbsp. Bread crumbs
2 tsp. Garlic powder 1 tbsp. Dried parsley Salt and pepper, to taste

111. Tandoori Chicken Legs

Cook time: 25 minutes / Serves 2

2 Whole chicken legs 4 fl. oz. Fatty Greek yogurt 2 tbsp. Olive oil ½ tsp. Cumin ½ tsp. Turmeric ½ tsp. Coriander 1/4 tsp. Cardamom
½ tsp. Cayenne pepper 1 tsp. Paprika Pinch of Nutmeg 1 Minced garlic clove ½ tsp. Fresh ginger 2 tbsp. Limejuice Salt and pepper, to taste

112. Baked Eggplant with Cheese

Prep. Time: 15 minutes / Serves 4

1 Large eggplant, sliced 1 big egg ½ cup Parmesan cheese, grated ¼ cup Pork dough
½ tbsp. Italian seasoning 1 cup low-sugar tomato sauce ½ cup Mozzarella, shredded 4 tbsp. Butter

113. Shrimp and Zucchini with Alfredo Sauce

Time: 5 minutes / Cook time: 15 minutes / Serves 6

8 oz. Shrimp peeled 2 tbsp. Butter ½ tsp Minced garlic 1 tbsp. Fresh lemon juice
2 Zucchini 2 oz. Heavy cream 3 oz. Parmesan cheese Salt and pepper to taste

114. Chicken Breasts in a Garlic-Cream Sauce

Time: 10 minutes/Serves 4

For the chicken: 2 Chicken bosoms 1 tbsp. Lemon juice 1/4 tsp. Stew powder 1 tsp. Crisp ground ginger 1 Minced garlic ½ tsp. Coriander powder ½ tsp. Turmeric 1 oz. Margarine

For the sauce: 4 oz. Overwhelming cream 3 tbsp. Squashed tomatoes 4 fl. oz. Chicken juices 1 Onion, diced 1 Garlic clove, minced 1/4 tsp. Bean stew powder 1 tsp. New ground ginger 1/4 tsp. Cinnamon

1. Cut the chicken bosoms into little pieces, at that point blend them in a bowl in with lemon juice, bean stew powder, ground ginger, cleaved garlic, coriander powder, turmeric, salt, and pepper.

2. Warmth 2 tablespoons of spread in a griddle over medium warmth, at that point include the onions and garlic and stew for 2 minutes or until fragrant.

3. Include chicken pieces and cook for 4-5 minutes. At the point when the chicken is white, include overwhelming cream, chicken juices, slashed tomatoes, and seasonings and blend well. Heat to the point of boiling, at that point decrease the warmth to least, spread and stew for 6-7 minutes.

4. On the off chance that you like the sauce thicker - evacuate the top and stew it to the ideal consistency.

5.Present with steamed broccoli or some other low-carb item to your taste.

Calories: 319. Fat: 21 g. Protein: 27 g. Carbs: 3.9

115. Salmon Filet with Cream Sauce

Time: 10 minutes

2 tbsp. Olive oil 3 Salmon filets 2 Garlic cloves, minced 1 cup substantial whipped cream 1 oz. Cream cheddar

2 tbsp. Escapades 1 tbsp. Lemon juice 2 tsp. Crisp dill 2 tbsp. Parmesan cheddar, ground

116. Hamburger Casserole with Cabbage and Cheese

Prep. Time: 15 minutes, Serves 8

2 lb. Cauliflower 8 oz. Relaxed cream cheddar 1 lb. Ground hamburger ½ Onion, diced 1 tbsp. Worcestershire Sauce 1 cup Shredded cracklings

1 Big egg 2-cup cheddar, ground 5 oz.

1.Cut the bacon, and afterward fry it in a hot skillet. Put it on a paper towel to retain abundance fat. Expel the vast majority of the fat from the container, and you will require just a couple of tablespoons.

2. Fry the onions until it is brilliant dark colored.

3. Include ground meat and fry well. Include the Worcestershire sauce and, if fundamental, seasonings. Move the blend to a huge bowl.

4. In a different bowl, blend the cabbage and cream cheddar, at that point whisk everything together utilizing a hand blender or blender. The consistency of
everything ought to resemble pureed potatoes. In the event that important, include flavoring.

117. Rich Spinach

Prep. Time: 10 minutes/Serves 4

2 tbsp. Spread 2 tbsp. Olive oil 1 Onion, minced

9 oz. New spinach 2 fl. oz. Cream cheddar 2 fl. oz. Substantial cream

1. Warmth the cream and olive oil in a skillet at medium-high temperature.

2. Include garlic and onions, and mix constantly for 2-3 minutes until delicate.

3. Include the spinach (a bunch at once) and fry until it wilts. Put in a fine strainer and crush the fluid.

4. Return the spinach to the container, season with pepper and salt, and include the substantial cream. Cook until rises in the cream.

5. Blend in with cream cheddar until it is totally dissolved, and the blend is thick and bubbly. Expel from warmth and serve. Calories: 277. Fat: 21 g. Protein: 9 g. Carbs: 7

118. Seared Cod with Tomato Sauce

Prep. Cook time: 20 minutes/Serves 4

A fish: 1 lb. (4 filets) Cod 1 tbsp. Spread 1 tbsp. Olive oil Salt and pepper, to taste

Tomato sauce: 3 huge egg yolks 3 tbsp. Warm water 8 oz. Margarine 2 tbsp. Tomato glue 2 tbsp. Crisp lemon juice

A fish:

1. Season the filets on the two sides. Note that the salt must be put at last, before cooking, so as not to consume the fish.

2. Pour olive oil over the base of the counter mesh skillet and turn on medium warmth. Include margarine. At the point when they start to sizzle, include cod filet and fry for a few minutes; at that point give it to the opposite side.

3. Tilt the container, gather the oil with a spoon, and dunk the fish in it. Keep cooking for another a few minutes.

119. Braised Beef in Orange Sauce

Prep. Time: 10 minutes/Cook time: an hour and a half/Serves 6

2 lb. Meat 3 cups Beef stock 3 tbsp. Coconut oil 1 Onion Peel and squeeze of 1 orange 2 tbsp. Apple vinegar 1 tbsp. Crisp thyme

2½ tsp. Garlic hacked 2 tsp. Ground cinnamon 2 tsp. Erythritol 1 tsp. Soy sauce Rosemary, perceptive, cove leaf, salt, pepper, to taste

120. Meatloaf

Prep. Time: 10 minutes/Cook time: an hour/Serves 8

1 lb. Ground meat ½ tsp. Garlic powder ½ tsp. Cumin 6 cuts cheddar

2 oz. Cut onions 2 oz. Green onions, hacked ½ cup Spinach ¼ cup Mushrooms

121. Keto Chili

Prep. Time: 10 minutes

Serves 6

2 lb. Youthful meat 8 oz. Spinach 1 cup Tomato sauce 2 oz. Parmesan cheddar 2 green ringer peppers 1 Onion

1 tbsp. Olive oil 1 tbsp. Cumin 1½ tbsp. Stew powder 2 tsp. Cayenne pepper 1 tsp. Garlic powder Salt and pepper, to taste

121. Meat Croquettes with Sausage and Cheese

Prep. Time: 10 minutes

/Serves 12

1 lb. Minced meat 1 Chorizo wiener 1-cup cheddar 8 fl. oz. Tomato sauce

3 oz. Destroyed pork skins 2 large eggs 1 tsp. Cumin 1 tsp. Stew

122. Eggplant with Bacon

Prep. Time: 10 minutes/Serves

1 tbsp. White wine 1 tbsp. Lemon juice 1 cup Parmesan cheddar, destroyed

1. Cut the bacon and fry it in a huge skillet over medium warmth.

2. At the point when the bacon is firm, haul it out of the skillet and spot it on a paper towel. Spare all the fat.
3. Strip and cut the eggplant. Cook it in bacon fat until it relaxes.

123. Cheesecake Keto-Cupcakes

Cook time: 20 minutes / Cook time: 15 minutes / Serves 12

4 oz. Almond flour 2 oz. Butter, melted 8 fl. oz. Soft cream cheese
2 Eggs 6 oz. Granulated keto sweetener 1 tsp. Vanilla extract
1. Heat the oven to 350 °F degrees. Layout the parchment 12 molds for muffins.

124. Chocolates with Berries

Cook time: 10 minutes / Cook time: 15 minutes / Serves 12

4 tbsp. Solid coconut oil 2 tbsp. Cocoa powder 1 tbsp. Erythritol or xylitol 1 tbsp. Liquid coconut oil
2 tbsp. Cocoa butter 1-cup Fresh berries mix Optional: grated unsweetened coconut or raw chopped nuts
1.Add solid coconut oil, cocoa butter, liquid coconut oil, salt, cocoa powder, and sweetener to taste in a saucepan, then stir over low heat until completely dissolved.

125. Keto Cookies with Raspberry Jam

Prep. Time: 10 minutes/Serves 12

3 cups of Almond flour 1/4 tsp Xanthan gum ½ tsp. Heating powder 4 oz. Delicate margarine 2 oz. Erythritol or another keto-accommodating sugar

1 tsp. Vanilla concentrates 1 Egg 3 tbsp. Raspberry jam/sugar free jam

1.Preheat the broiler to 370 °F degrees and spot a heating sheet with material paper.

2.Blend flour, thickener, preparing powder, and salt in a little bowl. Set aside.

3.In a bowl, beat the margarine and sugar until the mass gets breezy.

4.Include egg and vanilla concentrate.

5.Include the flour blend and blend well.

6.Gap the batter into 12 balls and spot on the readied heating sheet.

7.Snap on the focal point of each ball to make a treat. In the focal point of each spot 1/2 tsp. of jam.

8. Prepare treats for 10–12 minutes, until the edges are light brilliant dark colored.

9. Permit cooling until the jam solidifies.

Calories: 168. Fat: 16 g. Protein: 4 g. Carbs: 2

126. Chocolate Brownie in a Mug Prep. Time: 5 minutes / Serves 12

1 Big egg 2 tbsp. Almond flour ½ tsp. Baking powder 2 tbsp. Unsweetened cocoa powder
1 tbsp. Butter or coconut oil ½ tsp. Vanilla extract 1 tbsp. Stevia or keto-friendly sweetener of your choice
1. Oil one large cup or two small shapes. Put aside.
2. Add the ingredients and mix with a small whisk until smooth.
3. Pour the dough into the prepared form and place it in the microwave for about 1 minute (two servings) or 75 seconds per serving in a mug. Calories: 140. Fat: 9 g. Protein: 11 g. Carbs: 3

127. Lemon Blueberry Keto-Cakes

Prep. Time: 15minutes / Cook time: 22 minutes / Serves 12
Dough: 4 Eggs 3/4 cup Fatty coconut milk 1 tsp. pure vanilla extracts ½-cup Coconut flour 1½ tbsp. Xylitol 1 tsp. Baking powder ½ tsp. Xanthan gum 1/8 tsp. Pink Himalayan salt
3 tbsp. Herbal unsalted butter, melted 3/4 cup Fresh blueberries
Lemon icing: 1 Lemon, juice and zest 5 tbsp. Powdered (non-granular) stevia or xylitol
1. Preheat the oven to 370 °F degrees.
2. In a large bowl, mix the eggs, coconut milk, and vanilla.
3. Add coconut flour, xylitol, baking powder, xanthan gum, and salt, and beat well. Add melted butter and mix again.
4. Carefully add fresh blueberries.
5. Fill 12 cupcakes with dough, about half.

128. Chocolate Keto Fudge

Prep. Time: 5 minutes / Serves 12
½-cup Almond oil ½-cup Coconut oil 2 oz. Unsweetened cocoa powder
3 tbsp. Keto sweetener 1 tsp. Vanilla extracts 2 oz. Walnuts (optional)
1. Add coconut and almond oil, and cocoa powder in a blender, and beat until smooth.
2. Add vanilla, sweetener, and salt. If desired, add walnuts or other ingredients to your taste.

3.Add the mixture into a baking dish lined with parchment paper. Put it in the fridge until it is completely cool, then pull it out and cut it into 16 small squares.

129. Chocolate and Nutty Smoothies

Cooking time: 5 minutes/prep. Time: 5 minutes/Serves 2
1 tbsp. Nutella 1 banana
½ cup Milk 2 oz. Pecans
1.Cut the banana into cuts; include some milk and a tablespoon of chocolate glue and pecans (6–8 pieces).

2. For 1–2 minutes, prepared to smooth with chocolate chips.

130. Keto Taco

1.Warmth a grill to 375 °F. Put the foil on a preparing sheet and spread the bacon on it. Cook it for 15-20 minutes.

2. While bacon is cooked, put 3 oz. of mozzarella in a spotless dish and cook cheddar over medium warmth.
3. Trust that the cheddar will cook around the edges (around 2-3 minutes).
4. Utilize a couple of tongs and a wooden spoon to make a cheddar shell for tacos.
5.Do likewise with the remainder of your cheddar.

131. Keto Omelet with Goat Cheese and Spinach

Cooking time: 5 minutes/prep. Time: 10 minutes/Serves 1

3 Large eggs 1 Medium green onion 1 oz. Goat cheddar ¼ Onion
2 tbsp. Spread 2 cups Spinach 2 tbsp. Overwhelming cream Salt and pepper to taste
1.Cut the onion into long strips and fry it in oil until caramelized. Add the spinach to the container and fry a bit.
2. Expel the vegetables from the container — blend 3 huge eggs, cream, salt, and pepper together.
3. Empty the egg blend into the container and cook on medium warmth.
4. When the part of the omelet starts to boil, include a spoonful of spinach and onions to 1/2 omelet. Sprinkle with hacked goat cheddar.
5.At the point when the highest point of the omelet is prepared, you can serve. On the off chance that you like, enliven with onions on top.

132. Chicken and Cheese Quesadilla

Cooking time: 10 minutes/prep. Time: 15 minutes/Serves 4

For tablets: 6 Eggs 4 oz. Coconut flour 6 oz. Overwhelming cream ½ tsp.
Thickener Pink salt and pepper 1 tbsp. Olive oil for broiling
For the quesadilla: 4 oz. Cheddar destroyed 8 oz. Chicken bosom cooked
and destroyed 1 tbsp. Parsley, hacked (discretionary)
1. Blend in a bowl every one of the ingredients for the cakes, whisk well and
   let the batter represent 8-10 minutes.
2. Warmth the oil in a griddle over medium warmth and fry the tortillas
   for 2-3 minutes on each side or until cooked. Put aside to cool.
3. Warmth, a spotless frying pan over medium warmth, put one tortilla,
   sprinkle with cheddar, spread with a top, and hold up until the cheddar
   starts to dissolve. At that point, include slashed chicken meat, more
   cheddar, and covered with a subsequent level cake.

133. Vegan Scramble

Cooking time: 5 minutes/prep. Time: 15 minutes/Serves 5

The formula is anything but difficult to plan, yet delectable avocados,
tomatoes, and cheeses will lift your spirits and invigorate for extraordinary
deeds. 1 lb. Tofu cheddar 3 tbsp. Avocado oil 2 tbsp. Slashed onion 1½
tbsp. Nourishment yeast ½ tsp. Garlic powder ½ tsp. Turmeric ½ tsp. Salt
1-cup Spinach 3 Grape tomatoes 3 oz. Vegetarian Cheddar Cheese
1. Envelop the tofu by a few layers of paper or fabric towels, and delicately
   press some water. Set aside.
2. In a skillet over medium warmth, fry the cleaved onion in 1/3 tbsp.
   Avocado spread until onion is delicate and translucent
3. Spot the tofu in the dish and mix well with a fork.
4. Pour the rest of the oil and sprinkle with dry flavoring.
5. Fry the tofu over medium warmth, blending occasionally until the
   majority of the fluid has dissipated.
6. Include the spinach, dice the tomatoes and cheddar, and cook for a
   moment or until the spinach has blurred and the cheddar has softened.

7. Serve hot and store scraps in the cooler for a limit of three days.

134. Burger with Guacamole and Egg

Cooking time: 5 minutes/prep. Time: 10 minutes/Serves 1

Here and there in the morning, you truly need a delicious burger with
different flavors. Thusly, I have arranged for this superb formula.
Succulent meat, bright guacamole, an egg, and 10 minutes are all you have

to make the most of your most loved keto burgher. Everybody around will need the equivalent.

5 oz. Ground hamburger 4 Bacon, cuts 3 oz. Guacamole 1 Egg
1 tbsp. Olive oil (for fricasseeing) ½ tsp. Italian flavoring Salt and pepper to taste
1. In a little bowl, blend ground hamburger with Italian flavoring, salt, and pepper. Structure a little patty.
2. Put on cutting board 4 portions of bacon across, cutlet on top, and afterward fold bacon over it.
3. Warmth 1/2 tablespoons of olive oil in a griddle over medium warmth, include the cutlet in bacon and fry 3 minutes (or more, contingent upon thickness) on each side
4. Include the staying 1/2 tablespoons of oil to the dish and fry the egg, with the fluid yolk inside.
5. Put guacamole, a seared egg on a cutlet, and, if vital, season with salt and pepper. Cut down the middle and serve right away.
Calories: 443. Fat: 33 g. Protein: 32.5 g. Carbs: 2.4

135. Stuffed Avocado

Cooking time: 5 minutes/prep. Time: 10 minutes/Serves 1

1 Avocado hollowed and cut down the middle 1 tbsp. Spread, salted 3 large eggs
3 cuts of bacon cut into little pieces Salt and dark pepper, to taste
1. Wipe out the greater part of the avocado mash, leaving about 1.5 cm around.
2. Spot a huge skillet over low warmth and include margarine. While the spread is dissolving, break the eggs into a bowl and whisk them, including a touch of salt and pepper.
3. Spot bacon on one side of the container and fry for two or three minutes. On the opposite side, pour the egg blend and mix them routinely.
4. Eggs and bacon ought to be readied 5 minutes in the wake of adding eggs to the dish. In the event that you find that the eggs are cooked a little before the bacon, expel the fried eggs and spot them in a bowl.
5. Blend the bacon and fried eggs together, and afterward fill the avocado parts with the blend.
Calories: 500. Fat: 40 g. Protein: 25 g. Carbs: 11
Omelet with Mushrooms and Goat Cheese
Cooking time: 5 minutes/prep. Time: 10 minutes/Serves 1
3 Large eggs 2 tsp. overwhelming cream 3 oz. Cleaved mushrooms 1 tsp. Olive oil
2 oz. Disintegrated goat cheddar seasoning to taste Green onions for trimming
1. Warmth olive oil in a dish. Fry the mushrooms until delicate, about. 4 minutes.

2. While the mushrooms are being cooked, beat the eggs with overwhelming cream and a modest quantity of flavoring.
3. Pour the egg blend over the mushrooms and cook for around 2-3 minutes.
4. Include goat cheddar. Overlay the omelet into equal parts and keep cooking until the cheddar begins to soften.
5.Present with spring onions or another side dish to your taste.
Calories: 515. Fat: 39.5 g. Protein: 21 g. Carbs: 4.2

Fat Bombs

136. Neapolitan Fatty Bombs

Cooking time: 10 minutes/prep. Time: 15 minutes/Serves 24

½ cup Butter ½ cup Coconut oil ½ cup Sour cream ½ cup Cream cheddar 2 tbsp. Erythritol
25 drops liquid stevia 2 tbsp. Cocoa powder 1 tsp. Vanilla concentrate 2 medium strawberries
1. utilizing a blender, blend every one of the ingredients (aside from cocoa powder, vanilla, and strawberry) in a bowl.
2. Partition the blend between 3 dishes. Add cocoa powder to one, vanilla to another, and strawberries to third.
3. Empty the chocolate blend into the shape and spot in the cooler for 30 minutes. Rehash the procedure with vanilla and strawberry layers.
4. Presently put all stops for in any event 60 minutes.

137. Chocolate-Coconut Fat Bombs with Almonds

Cooking time: 5 minutes/prep. Time: 15 minutes/Serves 12

1 cup Coconut chips 3 tbsp. Fat coconut milk 3 tbsp. Coconut oil (softened) ½ tsp. Vanilla concentrate
4 oz. Chocolate chips, no sugar a spot of salt 2 oz. Keto-accommodating sugar 24 Almond, pieces
1.Put 2 tablespoons of softened coconut oil, coconut milk, sugar, coconut chips, vanilla concentrate, and salt in a little bowl.
2.Separation the blend into 12 servings and spot them on a preparing sheet with material paper. Put in the cooler for 5 minutes, at that point put on each fat bomb 1-2 things almonds.
3.Liquefy the chocolate chips together with 2 teaspoons of coconut oil in the microwave.
4.Expel the bombs from the cooler, pour every one of the chocolate blend and cool.

138. Spicy Fat Bombs

Cooking time: 5 minutes/prep. Time: 15 minutes/Serves 12

6 MCT powder scoops 10 Liquid stevia's, drops 1 tsp. Turmeric 1 tbsp. Dark sesame seeds Squeeze Chinese 5 Spice Blend a touch of dark pepper ½ tsp. Cinnamon 2½ fl. oz. Warm water

1. Blend all the dry ingredients in a little bowl.
2. Include warm water and blend until smooth.
3. Spread the blend equally more than 12 silicone molds, around 1 tbsp. L on each.
4. Put in the refrigerator, so the fat bombs are all around solidified. Continuously keep them solidified, else they will rapidly soften.

139. Espresso Fat Bombs

Cooking time: 5 minutes/prep. Time: 30 minutes/Serves 12

4 oz. Margarine 2 oz. Ghee spread (liquefied) 2 oz. Substantial cream 1 tbsp. Milk to your taste Double coffee
2 oz. Keto-accommodating sugar of your decision 1 tsp. Vanilla concentrate a spot of salt
1. Add all ingredients to a little nourishment processor and whip at rapid until vaporous.
2. Add sugar to taste.
3. Fill shape and refrigerate for 30 minutes (or more in the event that you wish)

140. Almond Coconut Fat Bombs

Cooking time: 5 minutes/prep. Time: 20 minutes/Serves 10

2 fl. oz. Almond oil 2 fl. oz. Coconut oil
2 tbsp. Cocoa powder 2 fl. oz. Erythritol, to your taste
1. Blend almond and coconut oil in a microwave dish.
2. Warmth the blend in the microwave for 30-45 seconds and blend until a homogeneous mass. Include erythritol and cocoa powder, and blend to finish the blend.
3. Empty the mass into scaled-down cupcake forms and refrigerate in the icebox.

141. Pumpkin Fat Spice Bombs

Cooking time: 5 minutes/prep. Time: 10 minutes/Serves 9

8 oz. Crude cashews 4 oz. Crude macadamia nuts 4 oz. Coconut chips 3 fl. oz. Pumpkin puree
2 tbsp. MCT oils 2 tsp. Cinnamon, ground 2 tsp. Ginger, and ground Neutral oil (avocado oil)

1. Put every one of the ingredients in a nourishment processor and blend to frame a mixture.
2. Delicately oil your hands with nonpartisan oil, for example, avocado oil. Utilizing a spoon, take about 3.5 - 4 oz. of the hitter into softly oiled hands and
structure a ball. Defer and rehash the procedure (around 9 "bombs" altogether).
3. Brighten fat bombs with appetizing coconut chips.
4. Such greasy bombs can be eaten promptly, or put away in an icebox/cooler.

142. Cheddar Fat Bombs in Bacon

Cooking time: 5 minutes/prep. Time: 20 minutes/Serves 20

8 oz. Mozzarella cheddar 4 tbsp. Almond flour 4 tbsp. Spread, dissolved 3 tbsp. Psyllium powder 1 Egg Salt, to taste

1 tsp. Dark pepper 1/8 tsp. Garlic powder 1/8 tsp. Onion powder 20 Bacon, cuts 1-cup oil or fat (for searing)

1. Microwave, a large portion of the cheddar for 45-60 seconds or until it softens and ends up clingy.
2. Warmth the margarine in the microwave for 15-20 seconds until totally softened. At that point, blend it with cheddar and egg.
3. Include psyllium husks, almond flour, and flavors. Blend again and spread out the mixture square shape.
4. Fill the square shape with the remainder of the cheddar and overlap it into equal parts (on a level plane), at that point down the middle (vertically).

5. Trim the edges and structure into a square shape. Cut 20 square pieces.
6. Wrap each bit of mixture with a bit of bacon, utilizing toothpicks to secure it.
7. Put each piece in bubbling oil and cook for 1-3 minutes.

143. Vegetable Salad with Bacon and Cheese

Cooking time: 5 minutes/prep. Time: 10 minutes/Serves 6

4 oz. Lettuce 3 oz. Spinach 2 oz. Wavy cabbage 6 cuts of cooked bacon 12 pcs. Grape tomato
1 Avocado stripped and cut 2 oz. Blue cheddar 3 tbsp. harsh cream 2 ½ tbsp. Mayonnaise
1. In a little bowl, blend the harsh cream and mayonnaise.
2. Blend with a large portion of the blue cheddar and put it in a safe spot.
3. In an enormous plate of mixed greens bowl, blend the rest of the ingredients.
4. Spread the serving of mixed greens into segments and spot the blue cheddar dressing on top.

144. A plate of mixed greens with Chicken Breast and Greens

Cooking time: 10 minutes/prep. Time: 30 minutes/Serves 2

2 tbsp. Pesto sauce 2 fl. oz. Balsamic vinegar 1 tsp. Olive oil 6 oz. Chicken bosom 4-cup spring greens
1 oz. New mozzarella ¼ Avocado, diced 6 Cherry tomatoes 1 tbsp. New basil for adornment
1. Set up the marinade by blending pesto, balsamic vinegar, and olive oil.
2. Put in a safe spot a segment of the marinade for the serving of mixed greens, and pour the staying chicken bosom. Refrigerate marinate for in any event
20 minutes.
3. Take the serving of mixed greens. Start with greens, at that point layered with crisp mozzarella, avocado, and tomatoes.
4. When the chicken is salted, heat the medium-sized iron, and afterward include a little olive oil.

145. Salmon Salad

Cooking time: 5 minutes/prep. Time: 10 minutes/Serves 2

2 Sheets of lettuce 6 leaves, Fresh basil, finely hacked ½ tsp. Garlic powder
1 tsp. Lemon juice
4 tbsp. Mayonnaise 5 oz. Salmon 1 oz. Red onion, hacked ½ Avocado, diced
2 tbsp. Parmesan cheddar, dice
1. Wash well and clean the lettuce leaves - they will fill in as plates.
2. Blend lemon juice hacked basil and garlic powder.
3. Include mayonnaise and blend well. Put in a safe spot.

4. Fill each "plate" of lettuce with half of the finely slashed salmon, and after that, avocado and onion rings.

146. Basic Cabbage and Egg Keto Salad

Cooking time: 10 minutes/prep. Time: 10 minutes/Serves 6

1 lb. Cauliflower flowers 4 oz. Keto mayonnaise 1 tsp. Yellow mustard 1½ tsp. Crisp dill Ground dark pepper and salt, to taste 2 oz. finely slashed dill

1 Celery stalk finely slashed 2 oz. Red onion slashed 1 tbsp. Salted keto cucumber, cleaved 6 Hard-bubbled eggs, hacked Paprika, for enhancement

1. Pour some water (about 2.5 cm) into an enormous pan, put 1 tsp. of salt and heat to the point of boiling. Include cauliflower and cook until prepared, from 8 to 10 minutes. Channel and put aside in an enormous bowl.
2. In a little bowl, blend mayonnaise, mustard, dill, a spot of salt and pepper. Put in a safe spot.
3. Pulverize 4 eggs and add to the cauliflower bowl. Cut the staying two eggs.

147. Light Pea and Green Onion Salad

Cooking time: 5 minutes/Cook time: 10 minutes/Serves

2 oz. Pea 2 tsp. Green onions ½ tsp. Soy sauce 2 tsp. Olive oil
½ tsp. Apple vinegar ½ tsp. Sesame oil ½ tsp. Sesame seeds Garlic powder, to taste.
1. Cut the green onions and peas corner to corner.
2. Blend the cleaved vegetables with the rest of the ingredients and blend. Spread and refrigerate for 2 hours.
3. Present with your preferred primary course - flame-broiled chicken, shrimps, salmon, and so on.

148. Keto-Salsa with Avocado and Shrimps

Cooking time: 10 minutes/Cook time: 10 minutes/Serves 4
8 oz. Stripped crude shrimp 1 tbsp. Olive oil 1 Lemon (juice) 1 Avocado, diced 1 Tomato, diced

1 Cucumber, diced 1/4 Onion, diced 2 oz. Cilantro, hacked Salt and dark pepper, to taste.
Season the shrimp with salt and pepper. Put the dish on medium-high heat and pour olive oil. When the oil has heated up, include the shrimp and fry one side for 2-3 minutes; at that point, go to the next.

149. Keto Salad Taco

Cooking time: 10 minutes/prep. Time: 20 minutes/Serves 4

1 lb. Ground hamburger from grass-bolstered meat 1 tsp. Ground cumin ½ tsp. Bean stew powder 1 tbsp. Garlic powder ½ tbsp. Pepper and Paprika Salt, to taste 4 cups Roman lettuce
1 Tomato 4 oz. Cheddar 4 oz. Cilantro 1 Avocado 4 oz. Most loved salsa 2 little limes 1 cup Cucumber, cut
1. Warmth a huge skillet over medium warmth and pour in some coconut oil. Include ground hamburger and all seasonings.
2. Blend well and fry until darker. Expel from warmth and cool somewhat.

Bites

150. Fast Keto Bread

Cooking time: 5 minutes/prep. Time: 10 minutes/Serves 10

2 tbsp. Almond flour ½ tbsp. Coconut flour 1/4 tsp. Preparing powder 1 Egg
½ tbsp. Ghee or spread 1 tbsp. Unsweetened milk of your choice
1. Blend all ingredients in a little bowl and speed until smooth
2. Oil a glass bowl or microwave dish with spread, ghee, or coconut oil.
3. Empty the batter into a form and spot in the microwave at high temperature for 90 seconds.
4. Cut and pour softened margarine as wanted. Calories: 45. Fat: 20 g. Protein: 7 g. Carbs: 3

151. Vitality Keto Bars with Nuts and Seeds

Cooking time: 10 minutes/prep. Time: 25 minutes/Serves 8

2 tbsp. Margarine or coconut oil 2 fl. oz. Without sugar 1 tsp. Vanilla concentrate 8 oz. Almond, hacked 8 oz. Crude macadamia nuts (finely hacked) 4 oz. Pumpkin seed
2 tbsp. Hemp seed 1-2 tsp. Keto sugar (if important) 4 oz. Low sugar chocolate chips ½ tsp. Coconut or spread, or ghee oil
1. Preheat the stove to 350 °F degrees and spread out a preparing dish with material paper. Put every one of the nuts and seeds in a huge bowl, and blend.
2. Soften spread or coconut oil with vanilla concentrate and syrup in a little pan over low heat.
3. Pour the hot blend over the nuts and seeds, and shake well. On the off chance that essential, include keto sugar (erythritol, stevia, and so forth.)

152. Low-Carb Flax Bread

Cooking time: 10 minutes/prep. Time: 15 minutes/Serves 8

1 oz. Almond flour 1½ Flaxseed 1 tsp. Heating powder Salt, to taste ½ tsp. Vinegar
4 drops liquid stevia 3 oz. Crude whisked egg 1 fl. oz. Coconut oil or margarine (liquefied)

153. Keto Mini Pizza

Cooking time: 5 minutes/prep. Time: 15 minutes/Serves 4

1 oz. Keto mayonnaise 1 tbsp. Crude eggs 2 tsp. Coconut oil softened 2 tsp. Almond flour
1 tsp. Coconut flour ½ tsp. Psyllium powder a spot of preparing powder and heating pop

154. Eggplant Keto Chips

Cooking time: 5 minutes/prep. Time: 20 minutes/Serves 4

2 fl. oz. Olive oil 1 Large eggplant (daintily cut) Sal and pepper to taste 1 tsp. Garlic powder ½ tsp. Dry basil ½ tsp. Dried oregano 2 tbsp. Parmesan cheddar

155. Cheddar Keto Sticks

Cooking time: 5 minutes/prep. Time: 15 minutes/Serves 3

3 Mozzarella cheddar sticks (cut down the middle) 4 oz. Almond flour 1 tbsp. Italian flavoring blends 2 tbsp. Ground parmesan cheddar
1 Big egg Salt, to taste 2 tbsp. Coconut oil 1 tbsp. Cleaved parsley
1. Put the cheddar in the cooler medium-term with the goal that it solidifies.
2. At that point, add coconut oil to a medium measured cast iron skillet and warmth it over low to medium warmth.
3. Break the egg into a shallow bowl and whisk well. In a different bowl, blend the almond flour, parmesan cheddar, and seasonings.

156. Chicken Keto Nuggets

Cooking time: 15 minutes/prep. Time: 6 hours/Serves 4

1 oz. Whipped egg whites 1 oz. Chicken bosom cooked and minced ½ oz. Coconut flour ½ tsp. Preparing powder

1 fl. oz. Olive oil ½ oz. Dissolved margarine 1 oz. Greasy 40% cream Salt, pepper, a touch of garlic powder, discretionary

157. Champignon Keto Burger

Cooking time: 5 minutes/prep. Time: 15 minutes/Serves 4

Ground meat ½ tsp. Garlic powder
½ tsp. Onion powder ½ tsp. Worcestershire Sauce 1 cheddar, cut 1 Slice of tomato 2 oz. Blended greens or arugula 1 tbsp. Low-sugar ketchup

1. Put the mushroom tops in a bowl or shallow plate and include olive oil, balsamic vinegar, and a large portion of the salt and pepper; marinate for at any rate 30 minutes.
2. Cook the bacon in a griddle over medium warmth until fresh, turning two or multiple times to broil each side equally. Put in a safe spot.

158. Feeding Beef Soup

Cooking time: 10 minutes/prep. Time: 30 minutes/Serves

1 lb. Ground meat 5 slices of bacon 1 tbsp. Olive oil 1 tbsp.
1-cup Shredded cheddar 2 fl. oz. Fat whipped cream 2 tsp. Psyllium powder 4 oz. Destroyed cheddar ½ oz. Hacked green onions ½-cup Sour cream

159. Keto Cheeseburger with Bacon

Cooking time: 10 minutes/prep. Time: 30 minutes/Serves 2

For the mixture: 8 oz. Mozzarella destroyed 4 oz. Almond flour 1 tbsp. Cream cheddar
For the filling: 5 oz. Ground hamburger 1 Slice of cheddar, cut into quarters 1 tsp. Mustard 4 Bacon, cuts 1 Whisked egg 1 tsp. Sesame 1 tsp. Olive oil Salad Leaves for Garnish (Optional)

160. Hot Keto Soup with Mushrooms

Cooking time: 10 minutes/prep. Time: 30 minutes/Serves 4

1 tbsp. Olive oil 1 Onion (daintily cut) 1 tbsp. Crisp ground ginger 3 Garlic, cloves (finely cleaved) 1 tsp. Chile 1 tbsp. Fish sauce
2 fl. oz. Soy sauce 2 fl. oz. Rice vinegar 4 oz. Mushrooms (daintily cut) 4 hard-bubbled eggs 2-3 parcels of shirataki noodles 5-cup Bone stock

1. Empty oil into a huge pan and put on medium warmth. Include the onion and cook for 3-3 minutes until delicate.

2. Add the rest of the ingredients to the dish (with the exception of eggs and noodles) — Cook over low heat for 20-30 minutes.

161. Greek Keto Moussaka

Prep. Time: 10 minutes/Cook time: 30 minutes/Serves

For the filling: ½ chopped eggplant 10 oz. You have minced chicken 3 tbsp. Marinara sauce 1 Minced garlic ½ Chopped onion 1 tsp. Dried oregano 1 tsp. Paprika

½ tsp. Ground cinnamon 2 tbsp. Olive oil For the sauce: 3 tbsp. Overwhelming cream 3 tbsp. Cream cheddar 3 oz. Squashed cheddar 1 Minced garlic

1. Spread out a foil heating sheet. Cut the eggplants, put them on a preparing sheet, and pour olive oil. Prepare the eggplants for 5 minutes or until brilliant dark-colored.

2. Warmth olive oil in a griddle includes hacked onion, cleaved garlic, and fry until delicate. Include cleaved chicken and seasonings and fry until the meat is cooked. Include the marinara sauce, blend, and cook for an additional 3 minutes.

3. Blend a large portion of the squashed cheddar, cream cheddar, substantial cream, garlic, and salt in a pot and cook on low heat until the cheddar is liquefied and the sauce turns out to be thick and uniform.

162. Almond Pancakes with Shrimp and Cheese

Prep. Time: 10 minutes

Serves 8

1 lb. Shrimp cooked and cleaved 2 oz. Almond flour 1 Whisked egg 2 oz. Mozzarella, destroyed

3 tbsp. Parmesan cheddar, ground 1 tbsp. Crisp dill hacked 1½ tbsp. Olive or coconut oil, for fricasseeing Salt and pepper, to taste.

163. Heated Halibut Cheese Breaded

Cooking time: 10 minutes/prep. Time: 15 minutes/Serves 6

2 lb. Halibut (around 6 filets) 1 tbsp. Margarine 3 tbsp. Ground parmesan cheddar 1 tbsp. Bread scraps

2 tsp. Garlic powder 1 tbsp. Dried parsley Salt and pepper, to taste

164. Baked Chicken Legs

2 Whole chicken legs 4 fl. oz. Greasy Greek yogurt 2 tbsp. Olive oil ½ tsp. Cumin ½ tsp. Turmeric ½ tsp. Coriander 1/4 tsp. Cardamom

½ tsp. Cayenne pepper 1 tsp. Paprika Pinch of Nutmeg 1 Minced garlic clove ½ tsp. Crisp ginger 2 tbsp. Lime juice Salt and pepper, to taste

165. Prepared Eggplant with Cheese

Prep. Time: 15 minutes/Cook time: an hour/Serves 4

1 Large eggplant cut 1 big egg ½-cup Parmesan cheddar, ground 1/4-cup Pork batter
½ tbsp. Italian flavoring 1 cup low-sugar tomato sauce ½ cup Mozzarella, destroyed 4 tbsp. Spread

166. Shrimp and Zucchini with Alfredo Sauce

Cooking time: 5 minutes/prep. Time: 15 minutes/Serves 6

8 oz. Shrimp stripped 2 tbsp. Margarine ½ tsp Minced garlic 1 tbsp. Crisp lemon juice
2 Zucchini 2 oz. Substantial cream 3 oz. Parmesan cheddar Salt and pepper to taste

167. Chicken Breasts in a Garlic-Cream Sauce

Cooking time: 10 minutes/Cook time: 25 minutes/Serves 4

For the chicken: 2 Chicken bosoms 1 tbsp. Lemon juice 1/4 tsp. Bean stew powder 1 tsp. Crisp ground ginger 1 Minced garlic ½ tsp. Coriander powder ½ tsp. Turmeric 1 oz. Margarine
For the sauce: 4 oz. Substantial cream 3 tbsp. Squashed tomatoes 4 fl. oz. Chicken soup 1 Onion, diced 1 Garlic clove, minced 1/4 tsp. Stew powder 1 tsp. Crisp ground ginger 1/4 tsp. Cinnamon

168. Salmon Filet with Cream Sauce

Cooking time: 10 minutes/Cook time: 15 minutes/Serves 3

2 tbsp. Olive oil 3 Salmon filets 2 Garlic cloves, minced 1 cup heavy whipped cream 1 oz. Cream cheddar
2 tbsp. Tricks 1 tbsp. Lemon juice 2 tsp. Crisp dill 2 tbsp. Parmesan cheddar, ground

169. Meat Casserole with Cabbage and Cheese

Cooking time: 15 minutes/Cook time: 30 minutes/Serves 8

2 lb. Cauliflower 8 oz. Mollified cream cheddar 1 lb. Ground hamburger ½ Onion, diced 1 tbsp. Worcestershire Sauce 1 cup Shredded cracklings

1 Big egg 2-cup cheddar, ground 5 oz. Bacon Salt and pepper, to taste Extra side dish: cleaved onion

170. Rich Spinach

Cooking time: 10 minutes/Cooking time: 20 minutes/Serves 4

2 tbsp. Margarine 2 tbsp. Olive oil 1 Onion, diced 2 Garlic cloves, minced 9 oz. Crisp spinach 2 fl. oz. Cream cheddar 2 fl. oz. Substantial cream

171. Seared Cod with Tomato Sauce

Cooking time: 10 minutes/Cook time: 20 minutes/Serves 4

A fish: 1 lb. (4 filets) Cod 1 tbsp. Spread 1 tbsp. Olive oil Salt and pepper, to taste
Tomato sauce: 3 large egg yolks 3 tbsp. Warm water 8 oz. Spread 2 tbsp. Tomato glue 2 tbsp. Crisp lemon juice

A fish:

1. Season the filets on the two sides. Note that the salt must be placed ultimately, before cooking, so as not to consume the fish.
2. Pour olive oil over the base of the counter mesh skillet and turn on medium warmth. Include spread. When they start to sizzle, include cod filet and fry for a few minutes; at that point, give it to the opposite side.
3. Tilt the dish, gather the oil with a spoon, and plunge the fish in it. Keep cooking for another a few minutes.

Tomato sauce:

172. Braised Beef in Orange Sauce

Prep. Time: 10 minutes/Cook time: an hour and a half/Serves 6

2 lb. Meat 3 cups Beef soup 3 tbsp. Coconut oil 1 Onion Peel and squeeze of 1 orange 2 tbsp. Apple vinegar 1 tbsp. Crisp thyme 2½ tsp. Garlic hacked 2 tsp. Ground cinnamon 2 tsp. Erythritol 1 tsp. Soy sauce Rosemary, wise, cove leaf, salt, pepper, to taste

173. Meatloaf

Prep. Time: 10 minutes/Cook time: an hour/Serves

1 lb. Ground hamburger ½ tsp. Garlic powder ½ tsp. Cumin 6 cuts cheddar
2 oz. Cut onions 2 oz. Green onions slashed ½ cup Spinach ¼ cup Mushrooms.

174. Keto Chili

Cooking time: 10 minutes/Cook time: 30 minutes/Serves 6

2 lb. Youthful meat 8 oz. Spinach 1 cup Tomato sauce 2 oz. Parmesan cheddar 2 Green ringer peppers 1 Onion
1 tbsp. Olive oil 1 tbsp. Cumin 1½ tbsp. Stew powder 2 tsp. Cayenne pepper
1 tsp. Garlic powder Salt and pepper, to taste

175. Hamburger Croquettes with Sausage and Cheese

Cooking time: 10 minutes/Cook time: 30 minutes/Serves 12

1 lb. Minced hamburger 1 Chorizo frankfurter 1-cup cheddar 8 fl. oz. Tomato sauce
3 oz. Destroyed pork skins 2 large eggs 1 tsp. Cumin 1 tsp. Bean stew

176. Eggplant with Bacon

Cooking time: 10 minutes

Serves 2
1 lb. Bacon 1 lb. Margarine 2 Garlic cloves, ground
1 tbsp. White wine 1 tbsp. Lemon juice 1-cup Parmesan cheddar, destroyed.

177. Cheesecake Keto-Cupcakes

Cooking time: 10 minutes/Cook time: 15 minutes/Serves 12

4 oz. Almond flour 2 oz. Spread, dissolved 8 fl. oz. Delicate cream cheddar
2 Eggs 6 oz. Granulated keto sugar 1 tsp. Vanilla concentrate

178. Chocolates with Berries

Cooking time: 10 minutes/Cook time: 15 minutes/Serves 12

4 tbsp. Strong coconut oil 2 tbsp. Cocoa powder 1 tbsp. Erythritol or xylitol 1 tbsp. Fluid coconut oil
2 tbsp. Cocoa spread 1-cup Fresh berries blend Optional: ground unsweetened coconut or crude slashed nuts.

177. Keto Cookies with Raspberry Jam

Cooking time: 10 minutes/Cook time: 15 minutes/Serves 12

3 cups of Almond flour 1/4 tsp Xanthan gum ½ tsp. Heating powder 4 oz. Delicate margarine 2 oz. Erythritol or other keto-friendly sugar
1 tsp. Vanilla concentrates 1 Egg 3 tbsp. Raspberry jam/sugar-free jam

178. Chocolate Brownie in a Mug

Cooking time: 5 minutes/Cooking time: 10 minutes/Serves 12

1 Big egg 2 tbsp. Almond flour ½ tsp. Heating powder 2 tbsp. Unsweetened cocoa powder
1 tbsp. Margarine or coconut oil ½ tsp. Vanilla concentrate 1 tbsp. Stevia or keto-accommodating sugar of your decision

179. Lemon Blueberry Keto-Cakes

Cooking time: 10 minutes/prep. Time: 20 minutes/Serves 12

Batter: 4 Eggs 3/4 cup Fatty coconut milk 1 tsp. Unadulterated vanilla concentrate ½ cup Coconut flour 1½ tbsp. Xylitol 1 tsp. Heating powder ½ tsp. Thickener 1/8 tsp. Pink Himalayan salt
3 tbsp. homegrown unsalted spread, dissolved 3/4 cup Fresh blueberries
Lemon icing: 1 Lemon, squeeze, and get-up-and-go 5 tbsp. Powdered (non-granular) stevia or xylitol

180. Chocolate Keto Fudge

Cooking time: 5 minutes/prep. Time: 10 minutes/Serves 12

½-cup Almond oil ½-cup Coconut oil 2 oz. Unsweetened cocoa powder
3 tbsp. Keto sugar 1 tsp. Vanilla concentrates 2 oz. Pecans (discretionary)

181. Cheesecake Mint

Cooking time: 10 minutes/Cook time: 15 minutes/Serves 6 1½-cup Almond flour 2½ cup powdered erythritol 5 tbsp. Liquefied margarine 1 lb. delicate cream cheddar 15 Whole mint leaves 2 fl. oz. cup Heavy cream 6 oz. — low-carb dark chocolate 1/4 tsp. Mint concentrates.

182. Handcrafted Keto Mayo

Cooking time: 5 minutes/prep. Time: 10 minutes/Serves 12

6 fl. oz. Olive oil 4 fl. oz. Coconut oil 1 Egg 2 Egg yolks
1 tsp. Dijon mustard Pinch of salt and smoked paprika 3 drops Liquid Stevia.

183. Handcrafted Sambal Sauce

Cooking time: 5 minutes/prep. Time: 30 minutes/Serves 10

1 Onion 2 tsp. Stew peppers dried 3 tbsp. Low-sugar ketchup 2 tbsp. Coconut oil Salt, to taste

184. Low Carb Ketchup

Time: 5 minutes/Cook time: 5 minutes/Serves 10

3/4 cup Tomato glue 2 tbsp. Apple juice vinegar 2 tsp. Keto sugar Pinch of salt

185. Dutch Keto Sauce

Cooking time: 5 minutes/Cook time: 5 minutes/Serves 10

6 Egg yolks 1-drop Worcestershire sauce 1-drop Low carb hot sauce 1 Lemon, juice A squeeze of salt and ground dark pepper 8 oz. Margarine

186. Tapenade Keto Sauce

Cooking time: 5 minutes/prep time: 5 minutes/Serves 8

1 cup Black olives in saline solution 1 oz. Tricks 4 fl. oz. Blend Olive and Avocado oils 2 Garlic, cloves
3 tbsp. Lemon juice 2 tsp. Apple juice vinegar 1-cup Fresh basil 1-cup Fresh parsley ½ tsp. Dark pepper

187. Meat Keto Sauce

Cooking: 5 minutes/Cook time: 5 minutes/Serves 8

1 Shallot 4 Garlic, cloves ½-cup Cilantro ½-cup Parsley 1 Lemon juice
3 tbsp. Red wine vinegar 2 tsp. Squashed red pepper Pinch of salt and dark
pepper ¼-cup Olive oil

188. Speedy Pickled Keto Vegetables

Cooking time: 5 minutes/Cook time: 5 minutes/Serves 10 1½-cup Filtered
water 1½-cup Apple juice vinegar 1½ tbsp. Pink Himalayan salt

OTHER

189. Keto Bulletproof Coffee

Each keto dieter ought to have this keto espresso formula under control. It is a straightforward blend of only three ingredients: espresso, grass bolstered spread and MCT oil powder.

Blend every one of the three out of a blender to make a superbly foamy and invigorating latte. At that point, do not hesitate to zest up your keto espresso with increases to make each cup one of a kind.

190. Keto Brunch Spread

There are just three ingredients in this keto early lunch spread formula — eggs, asparagus, and bacon —yet it's extravagant enough for informal breakfast with the organization and simple enough for an end of the week in with your boo.

191. Immaculate Keto Avocado Breakfast Bowl

You most likely as of now have every one of the five ingredients expected to prepare this keto avocado breakfast bowl formula. What's more, it is so natural and fasts you can make it before you run out the entryway for work or school in the first part of the day.

192. Baked Pesto Chicken

This baked pesto chicken formula from Joy Filled Eats just requires an outing to the market for chicken bosoms, mozzarella, and basil pesto. You can either make your pesto without any preparation to control the carbs or discover a premade low-carb alternative at the store, contingent upon how much time you have.

193. Fiery Keto Cheese Crisps

At the point when you are sneaking for snacks and maintaining a strategic distance from chips, have a go at preparing a clump of zesty keto cheddar crisps for the ideal sans carb chomp.

6. Cloud Bread: 4-Ingredient, Low-Carb Bread

Did you know it just takes four ingredients to bring feathery keto cloud bread into your life? For whatever time that you have eggs, cream cheddar, salt, and a touch of cream of tartar, you are good to go.

194. Speedy RECIPES USING KETO PANTRY STAPLES

At the point when you are low on schedule or there is a storm or snowstorm outside, it is what is in your storeroom that isolates the keto novices from the genuine keto MVPs.

That is the reason a well-supplied keto washroom is worth twofold the cash you spend filling it.

195. Keto Oatmeal: 5-Minute Low-Carb N'Oats

Never miss the warm solace of oats on a nippy morning since you are in ketosis. This keto N'Oats formula joins flax, hemp, and chia seeds with coconut chips, almond milk, and a scoop of vanilla MCT oil powder.

196. Bacon, Egg and Cheese Breakfast Casserole

A well-supplied keto washroom likewise stretches out to your refrigerator.

You ought to consistently have bacon, ham or frankfurter, eggs, and cheddar around when you are on a keto diet because:

• The ingredients are cheap and last a respectable measure of time in your refrigerator

• There are unlimited approaches to set them up together.

• All cooking strategies are moderately quick and simple.

• They are stuffed with protein and great fat and very low in the carb office.

197. Meat-Lover Pizza Cups

Being on a keto diet implies you likely have unfulfilled pizza yearnings and a ton of meat in your ice chest.

198. Chocolatey Keto Nut Butter Cups

A chocolatey nutty spread cup you can make in the microwave with staples like margarine, overwhelming cream, Perfect Keto Nut Butter, and unsweetened chocolate? Truly, if it is not too much trouble.

When you just have 30 minutes to chow down and a little lunch cooler to fit it all in? You can either discover keto-accommodating suppers at the drive-through or pack one of these keto lunch recipes.

199. Simple Keto Chicken Salad

At the point when you start cluster preparing all your keto suppers for the week, you may wind up with an overabundance of chicken. This simple keto chicken plate of mixed greens is the solution to your extra chicken's reprise execution.

200. Spinach-Mozzarella Stuffed Burgers

Bugless burgers are everything on keto because they are so natural and adaptable. Move on from fixing your burgers with cheddar to stuffing them with this raised at this point straightforward spinach-mozzarella stuffed burgers formula from The Iron You.

NATURAL REMEDIES

Table of Contents

Medical Disclaimer

The information in this book is not to be used as medical advice. The information presented should be used in combination with guidance from your physician. All rights reserved. No part of this publication or the information in it may be quoted from or reproduced in any form by means such as printing, scanning, photocopying, or otherwise without prior written permission of the copyright holder.

The effort has been made to ensure that the information in this book is accurate and complete; however, the author and the publisher do not warrant the accuracy of the information, text, and graphics contained within the book due to the rapidly changing nature of science, research, known and unknown facts, and internet. The Author and the publisher do not hold any responsibility for errors, omissions, or contrary interpretation of the subject matter herein. This book is presented solely for motivational and informational purposes only.

Introduction

Herbal Medicine

The term *herbal medicine* seems pretty straightforward. It's herbs that are used as medicine. No surprise there, but what makes these herbs medicinal? And how did we learn to use them? We'll also cover the benefits of using herbs to heal.

A lot of plants can be used medicinally. From the roots to the treetops, each part of a plant can be useful in healing different ailments. Plants contain chemicals that have positive, negative, or neutral effects on the body. For example, most parts of deadly nightshade (belladonna), as the name might suggest, are very toxic and were used as a poison in folklore. However, the leaves and roots of the plant can be used as a muscle relaxant and for peptic ulcers. So, this plant has both positive and negative aspects. Despite how interesting it sounds, do not take deadly nightshade unless it's prescribed to you. An overdose can be fatal. The plants that have positive aspects if taken in the right dosage are those that are used for herbal medicine and are the basis for modern medicine.

Beyond simply plants grown for herbal use, many plants we eat are also effective for herbal medicine. If you've ever lived outside of Western nations, you may be familiar with fruits and vegetables that are eaten for specific illnesses. Papaya, for example, is not just a delicious fruit for snacking on but is also used for deworming, digestive issues, and healing wounds. In the US, foods that double as medicine include oats, lemons, onions, and garlic. These are foods easily, and inexpensively found in grocery stores across the US. They each have beneficial uses and are great to have on hand. So herbal medicine can include edible plants and herbal plants.

History of Herbal Medicine

Herbal medicine is ancient, and let's just say we wouldn't have gotten where we are as a species without it. If it weren't for herbal medicine, our life span would be 30 years or less. However, the use of herbal medicine helped us heal ailments and live longer. A lot of people will say this is due to modern medicine, but realistically, most people around the world were not using modern medicine until recently. Instead, they relied on herbal medicine. Even now, in areas where modern medications are too expensive, inaccessible, too dangerous, or no longer useful, herbal medicines are the go-to for most communities.

Herbal medicine can be traced back to ancient times. And when I say ancient, I don't mean 100 years ago. Herbal medicine can be found in folklore, burial sites, and religions dating back 60,000 years! The written content of herbs precedes most Western knowledge. The Egyptians and Indians have written lore about herbal medicine from 1500 BCE. All this folklore evolved over the centuries to become traditional medicine in different regions. In the West, herbal medicine evolved from the writings of Greek physicians, but by that point, China and India had already established herbal treatments that are still used today. So, when you practice herbal medicine, you are continuing the traditions of our ancestors and reinforcing the bond between humans and nature.

Today, herbal medicine is having a resurgence in the West, though it hasn't disappeared from other areas of the world. In countries where malaria is a frequent disease, many communities use herbal remedies when more modern medicine fails or isn't available. Unfortunately, modern medicine, while amazing, is also starting to fail. Many of our diseases are adapting to modern medicine and are becoming resistant to them. In cases like this, herbal medicine can be used to help. Using more herbal medicines, instead of relying on synthetic ones, can help to ensure that diseases are treated, even if they are medicine-resistant.

Benefits of Herbal Medicine

Beyond helping in drug-resistant cases, herbal medicine has a number of additional key benefits.

If you live in the US, you may be familiar with the expense of healthcare. It can be draining, and if you don't have health insurance, you may have to pay a lot out of pocket for medicine. Which, to be honest, is ridiculous since some of these medications are necessary for our lives. So, while modern synthetic medications can be expensive, herbal remedies are not. They are usually pretty cost-effective, and if you grow them yourself, they can be inexpensive. For example, you can purchase a growing calendula plant for probably $4 a plant. However, I can purchase a packet of calendula seeds for about $1.00. Since I can grow over 30 plants with the packet, that's a steal at about $.03 [LA1] per plant. Calendula is one of the most beneficial plants in herbal medicine. So, herbal remedies can be incredibly inexpensive in comparison to modern medicines.

If money isn't your concern, then you may be interested in the fact that herbal remedies are better for your body. Often, the modern medication causes side effects that can be pretty severe. We've all seen those commercials where they advertise a medication and then promptly, and very quickly, go through all the possible side effects. A lot of them are...intense. And knowing that your allergy medication can increase your likelihood of death is really off-putting. Herbal remedies can help with this.

3

While they can have some side effects, so long as you are following the correct dosages, it's rare for the side effects to be severe.

Another downside to modern medicine, but a benefit of herbal remedies, is that modern medications can be addictive. In fact, many synthetic pain medications are known to be highly addictive because of their close relation to drugs like cocaine and heroin. A single dose of pain medication can be addictive. Herbal remedies are not addictive for the most part, unless, of course, you choose to convert them into an addictive drug. After all, opium is highly addictive and comes from the poppy plant. However, it's an effective pain reliever and cold remedy if used in the right doses and preparation.

Caution

While herbal medicine is very effective and promising, there are, of course, some warnings that come with it.

Herbal medicine must be used precisely in order to control any potential negative effects. They have to be well-known and understood before being taken. If you don't know how they will affect you, whether they are toxic or not, or what ailments they remedy, then you shouldn't take them. You have to know the herbs you're taking and why you are taking them.

You also have to use quality herbs for remedies, or else they may be ineffective. At worst, they could be contaminated and harmful to your health. So, if you are choosing to take herbal remedies, do so only after you are knowledgeable about the herbs you want to take. Otherwise, only take herbal remedies prepared by registered herbalists who have had extensive training.

Chapter 1. Reasons to Consider Alternative and Herbal Medications

protect their health. In fact, the World Health Organization (WHO) approximates that about 80% of the entire world population includes herbal medicines as part of their health treatment.er balremedies continue toincreaseinpopularity. More and more people choose to benefit from these natural remedies to treat their ailments and

Here you will discover four (4) of the incredible things that herbal remedies can do. You may haven't yet known about some of these things, and your physician may never tell you about the other things.

More Affordable Treatment

Using herbs as natural remedies enable you to save your hard-earned money. Saving money may not be possible with pharmaceutical medicines, given their typically high cost. Aside from being the more affordable solution for ailments, botanical remedies are also equally effective compared to drug-based medications.

The Harvard Medical School recognizes the ability of botanicals to heal. In fact, it has published a _special health report_ on how to treat common pain conditions without using drugs or surgery. Results from several studies and research likewise show that plant-based medications work well with the body systems.

Safer Treatment than Drugs

Herbs and other natural remedies are safer treatment than drug-based medicines. Typically, herbal medicines do not carry side effects because of their natural composition. Drugs, on the other hand, contain active ingredients that interfere with the body systems; hence, the side effects.

Side effects of pharmaceutical medicines often occur (a) when you start taking the medication, (b) change the dosage either to lower it or to strengthen it, and (c) when you stop taking your medicine(s). In contrast, the side effects that may happen with herbal treatments are normally attributable to the improper use of the medication.

Potency Similar to Pharmaceuticals

At first glance, herbal medicines may not be as potent as pharmaceutical medicines when it comes to comparing their dosage. For instance, a cup of tea of willow bark (naturally containing aspirin and works as a pain reliever) is weaker in dosage than the standard dosage of pharmaceutical aspirin.

However, instead of looking at the dosage comparison, look at the effects of these medications. If taking a cup of willow bark can suffice to relieve your pain, why risk your general health to the typical side effects of pharmaceutical medicines? Keep in mind a general rule in medication: Start taking your medicine with the lowest dosage possible.

More Effective Treatment for Chronic Conditions

Unless your medical condition needs urgent intervention or treatment, herbal remedies are usually more effective than drug-based medications. With chronic conditions, treatment may require a longer period involving repeated use of the medication(s). This could mean greater risks of side effects with pharmaceuticals.

Botanicals, on the other hand, have no side effects or minimal side effects only. As mentioned earlier, the side effects typically occur only with improper use or dosage. Herbs contain natural chemicals that can sufficiently address chronic health conditions without the risk of side effects.

Chapter 2. Precautions to Ensure You Use Herbal Medicine Safely and Usage Target

Choose the right things? What would be the best kind of preparation to create, and what do we need to make that happen? You'll find that there are a lot of things and bits of information that can make the processes easier and less intimidating. Erbalmedi cinemakingisanincredi blyfulfillingskill topossess. Beforewedigin,there are some details and preparations to think about. How do we

Sourcing Medicinal Plants

Purchasing herbs may seem difficult, but there are a few simple things you can do to ensure that you're getting good-quality plant medicine. The ideal situation is to seek out an herb shop where the person behind the counter knows where the herbs came from and can help you decide. Be aware that, legally, they cannot prescribe or diagnose.

Herb shops aren't always available, but there are some very good places to source herbs online. I recommend that (at least at first) you purchase in smaller quantities, so you can see if the herb is one that works for you. If you have the space, growing herbs is also a fantastic way to access high-quality, fresh herbs, so go for it!

Common Preparations to Buy

It's easy to purchase good herbal medicine. In the list that follows, I've provided the most common herbal preparations you can find to buy. I've also marked those that are easy to make at home with an asterisk. (And you can surely make the rest at home, but they may require more instruction, study, or attention to detail.) Whether you purchase or DIY comes down to your budget and how much time, energy, and motivation you've got. When you're feeling blue, it may be easier to purchase your herbs online and have them delivered to your door, and know that's a great option.

Teas

- Tinctures (easy but need to sit for a few weeks)

- Fresh or dried individual herbs

Syrups

- Capsules or lozenges

- Balms and salves

Lotions

- Thin cream lotion

- Herbal water-infused lotion

Soaps

- Bath teas and soaks

Elixirs

- Herbal vinegar (easy but may need to sit for a few weeks)

- Infused honey (easy but may need time to infuse)

- Seasonings for food

Red Flags to Avoid

Steer clear of herbs that have lost their color—and, by extension, their vitality. The dull color indicates that they've been sitting around, and age, as well as poor storage practices, will diminish the plant's medicinal properties. Never purchase any kind of herbal product from a gas station or convenience store because they're selling a trend and don't know anything about it. Instead, go directly to herb sellers who are only working with herbs and herbal products rather than unfamiliar, random web stores.

Protecting Plants at Risk

Years ago, people in rural communities commonly made their livings by foraging and collecting wild plants for drug companies. This is still done, but more herbs are cultivated. However, there are still several plants that thrive and are more potent growing in the wild. These plants face many threats. Loss of habitat, use of herbicides, and fewer and fewer pollinators are part of the problem, and as more people become interested in herbs, overharvesting is a huge issue. Wild ginseng, goldenseal, and trillium are rare sights because they're worth money. Sandalwood and Palo Santo are popular scents, the plants of which are becoming few and far between. Here's how you can help keep these herbal allies from becoming threatened.

- Learn alternatives to at-risk herbs.

- Never use more than you need.

- If you choose to harvest a wild plant, take no more than 10 percent of a stand, leaving seeds behind. If there is only one stand, take nothing.

- Consider planting some endangered plants on your property to replace what you use.

- Join and contribute to United Plant Savers (unitedplantsavers.org) to be aware of the plants that are at risk.

There are people who still sell these plants and products made from them. Do not hesitate to ask about the origin. As an example, white sage is at risk, so I grow it and distill it for the hydrosol, taking nothing from the wild. There will be times when it is reasonable to use one of these herbs, but be mindful of their status and buy or use only what you really need. Don't waste it. It is so much better to learn about and use plants that are growing abundantly around you.

Best Practices and Safety Precautions

A safe and respectful approach to herbal medicine will lead to rich and fulfilling experiences.

Best Practices

I've learned the following best practices and found that they make herbalism feel like a lifestyle. (Which, as you may be coming to realize, it is!)

- Choose one herb when there is no urgent need to use it, and really get to know it. Note how it makes you feel. Then do the same with another single herb. That way, you can begin to understand how herbs affect you. If you make or buy a blend and then have a reaction, there's no way to know which herb caused it. If the blend works like magic, again, it will be a mystery. As you find your own allies, it will be easier and easier to discern what you need.

- Find a few people nearby who are interested in learning about herbs. Gather in a kitchen and try blending teas, making salves, or whatever you've wanted to try. Take field guides out into the woods and work together to identify plants. Each person brings some knowledge, whether they know it or not, and it's fun. Join some online groups and learn from the discussions. I still learn new things all the time from both of those sources.

- Make small batches of herbal medicine. I love to make 4-ounce batches of tinctures when working with a new herb and never make more than a pint. An ounce or two of a tea blend is usually plenty.

- Choose a preparation that you will actually use. Something that sits in a jar because it's unpleasant to take isn't helping at all. Capsules get a pretty bad rap because herbs are thought to be more easily absorbed in teas, tinctures, vinegar, and the like, but for many people, they're the most convenient method of taking herbs. The best way to take herbs is the way you will actually take them. They only work if they are used.

- If an herb shop salesperson attempts to add several more products to your purchase, be wary. Herbs can get expensive. It's frustrating to have a cupboard full of bottles and jars that didn't work and cost a paycheck.

Instead, get one or two items at a time unless a
- practitioner has recommended them. Keep in mind that
in medicine, pharmacists don't diagnose or prescribe,
and physicians don't sell drugs. That is to protect
patients and consumers. The lines aren't that clear in
herbalism, so it's something to consider.

Safety Precautions

Before long, working safely with herbs will become second nature, but
here are some tips to help you establish good habits:

- Always label everything. You will not remember what's in
that amber bottle next spring, and you will need to throw
it out, and that is very sad. There is a bottle of tincture
and a jar of some kind of infused oil downstairs right now
that I have to throw out for this very reason. (Yes, I still
overestimate my memory sometimes.) Labeling for
personal use should include the ingredients, the date,
what it is, and why it was made.

- Wash bottles and jars in hot soapy water prior to use.
Running them through the dishwasher is great, too.

- Small batches mean that there is less chance of spoilage.
It's better to make enough for a week or two and then
make it again than to make too much and have it gone
bad. Alcohol and vinegar are very good preservatives, so
products made with them are very safe, but it is still best
to use them up.

- Just because herbs are natural, it doesn't mean they are
harmless—if they weren't powerful, they couldn't help
you! Less is usually more, so work up to larger doses. Be
sure of the herb. It's always good to check more than one
source of information.

- Honey, especially raw honey—which is generally
preferred—should not be given to children younger than
one-year-old. Their digestive systems are not mature
enough to process Clostridium, a bacterium often found
in honey that can turn into botulism in infants.

11

Tools, Equipment, and Ingredients

Happily, there are very few things needed that you don't already have in the kitchen. Over the years, I've accumulated some really cool herb tools, but they arrived either as gifts or from a yard sale or thrift store. The hunt was half the fun! Some people enjoy going all out and getting the fancy equipment, but it can also be done inexpensively.

Essential Tools and Equipment

I started on a shoestring and can honestly say that with a whisk, measuring spoons and cups, a tea strainer, and some jars, it is possible to make just about everything you'll find in this book. There are some other items that come in handy and make the process more enjoyable, and it's much easier to work with some good tools.

- Whisk to combine wet or dry ingredients

- Containers: jars, bottles, and waterproof bag (feel free to reuse all glass bottles and jars of a reasonable size; just wash and sterilize them first)

- Fine-mesh strainer or 8-inch to 12-inch squares of cloth from worn-out T-shirts, sheets, or flannel

- Mixing bowls in a few different sizes or a 1- or 2-quart glass measuring cup

- A few dark glass dropper bottles in various sizes—1-ounce, 2-ounce, and 4-ounce—to hold finished and strained liquids

- Small jars for salves and lip balms

- Labels

- Permanent marker: something that won't smudge if it gets wet

- Some other items that are quite possibly already in your kitchen or that you will want to keep an eye out for as your herbal adventures continue:

- Coffee grinder for powdering herbs (a mortar and pestle may look cool, but the coffee grinder will save you time and your wrists)

- 5-by-8-inch muslin bags: great for making half gallons of tea or straining tinctures or oils

- Electric teapot to heat water quickly (I use mine nearly every day)

- 1-quart slow cooker: good for decoctions of roots and barks for tea or for infusing oils

- Blender: helps combine any sort of dry ingredients or chops up fresh herbs for tincturing

- Pipettes: long, disposable droppers.

Chapter 3. Herbal Remedies for Children

There are many easy to grow herbs that make wonderful remedies for children. You can even get children to grow their own medicine! Base your children's herb garden on their age.

In the garden, choose herbs that will be colorful, such as calendula. Lamb's ears are fuzzy and fun for children - they are soft and can be used as absorbent bandages for small scratches. The little ones love to stroke them. Older children love to learn that it is called the "toilet paper factory." Mullein is also referred to as a "toilet paper factory."

Plant a variety of herbs that smell and taste great. Lemon balm and other members of the mint family are always popular with children. Fortunately, these herbs are all very easy to grow and can tolerate even the loving care of even the smallest children.

Use your herb garden as a springboard to teach kids about nature, create nutritious meals, and make fun crafts. The best herbal medicine for children and everyone is to play with the herbs that grow in the earth. Even an herb garden by a window can introduce children to the natural world.

Here are some of the best herbs for kids. By the way, all these herbs also help adults.

Dill (Anethum Graveolens)

Dill is the most common flavoring for making pickles. It is also an exceptional remedy for children.

I grew the best crop of dill in a large tub this year - it was one of the shorter varieties, so it didn't bend, and the seed heads kept coming!

Try to squeeze the finely cut foliage and seed heads between the pages of an old phone book for herbal crafts. It's easy and fun.

In medicine, I use dill as an exceptional remedy for colic or any respiratory congestion. It is very safe. Nursing mothers can drink an infusion of the foliage or make a decoction of the seeds to relieve babies with colic. The root can also be decocted, although that's not something I do. The seeds are convenient, and the foliage is tasty.

Incorporate dill into some of your bread recipes. It's a rye bread classic. Dill is also a great flavor when used in stews.

Catnip (Nepeta Cataria)

Catnip can drive your cat crazy, but it's one of the best herbs for calming and soothing children. Unfortunately, kids don't agree with cats and don't believe catnip tastes good. It has a strange bitter flavor, so you need to mask its taste with other herbs or make a tasty preparation, like syrup or candy.

Catnip is my first choice for soothing discomfort caused by teething or colic. It's very relaxing and makes a great lukewarm bath to lower a fever.

Catnip can be used to relieve childhood diarrhea. I combine it with dill and blackberry leaves for this problem.

For minor hyperactivity, try combing catnip with lemon balm, passionflower, or chamomile.

Calendula (Calendula Officinalis)

Calendula is also known as 'pot marigold.' It is an edible flower. If you grow your own calendula, notice how sticky the flowers are: they're full of emollient healing compounds that improve wound healing and protect delicate skin.

My stepdaughter makes an ointment with calendula flowers infused in olive oil on the windowsill. She uses the wonderful balm for her little girl's buttocks. Thanks to her excellent care and this wonderful ointment, my granddaughter has never had a diaper rash. It's quite an accomplishment! The oil can also be used to relieve earaches, as long as there is no ruptured eardrum.
Calendula's bright orange and yellow flowers are packed with skin-healing benefits phytochemicals that help cells repair themselves, fight fungal growth, and provide antiseptic protection against bacteria.

This herb can be used to relieve shingles and minor burns. As a hot poultice or compress, it will reduce the pain of an earache.

It also reduces external and internal inflammation. It has been used to treat ulcers, reduce fevers, and relieve menstrual cramps and indigestion.

Calendula, when combined with chamomile, makes an excellent hair rinse, especially for blonde hair.

Making herbal remedies for kids is fun, inexpensive, and safe. Try to prepare remedies in advance so that you have them on hand if your child has a "boo-boo" or develops some of the common childhood complaints.

Dill and Apple Lollipops

These are easy to make and are great for stomach aches and loose stools. To make them rich in vitamin C, add 2 teaspoons of rose hips when you remove the pan from the heat. You can also add 2 teaspoons of elderberries before heating the final juice in order to boost your child's immune function.

Ingredients:

- Frozen pop molds

- 2 cups of organic apple juice

- 2 teaspoons dill seeds

Instructions:

1. Crush the seeds in a mortar and pestle or coarsely grind in a coffee grinder. Simmer the seeds in the juice for 20 minutes, covered, over low heat. Remove from the stove.

2. Cool slightly. Filter and compost the seeds. Pour the juice into soft drink molds. Freeze until firm. The yield varies depending on the size of the mussels.

Baby Bottom Balm

No baby should ever have a diaper rash. Cleanse your baby's skin with each diaper change and allow the skin time to air out.

Use a thin layer of this ointment to prevent stool and urine from irritating sensitive skin. This ointment is also helpful in soothing minor scrapes and cuts. Do not use ointments on a fresh burn; rather, use this after the healing has started.

Ingredients:

- 1 oz. calendula flowers

- 1 cup olive oil

- 2 tbsp. beeswax, grated

Instructions:

1. Place the herbs in a clean pot. Cover with oil. The oil should cover the grass by about an inch. Blanket. Place in a warm location, such as on a sunny window sill. Shake vigorously at least once a day. Let sit for two weeks.

2. Filter the flowers with a fine mesh colander, cheesecloth, or coffee filter and add them to your compost pile. Make sure all parts of the plant are filtered.

3. Combine beeswax and infused oil in a double boiler and heat until the wax melts. Stir. Continue to heat for an additional minute. Pour into clean, used baby jars or other containers. Let cool. Apply the lids.

4. The yield is 1 cup. This ointment does not need to be refrigerated because of the beeswax.

Catnip Bath Fever Remedy

It is an excellent fever reducer. If your child has a condition that causes skin irritation, you can put two cups of oatmeal in a clean stocking or sock and add it to the tub to soothe your child's skin.

Ingredients:

- 1 cup of catnip

- 4 cups of boiling water

Instructions:

1. Pour boiling water over the catnip. Blanket. Filter the herbs and compost them.

2. Let the catnip infusion cool to room temperature.

3. Add it to a lukewarm bath (the bath should not be hot or cold).

4. Let your child soak in the tub for up to 20 minutes.

Nature's Medicinal Balloons for Colds, Ear Infections, Flu and Other Respiratory Ailments

This recipe hides the taste of less flavorful herbs and is traditionally and historically used to reduce fever and treat infections. I use it when children have respiratory illnesses. They are very delicious and full of nutrients.

Ingredients:

- 1/4 cup almond butter

- 1/4 cup honey

- 2 tbsps. echinacea root, powdered

- 1 tbsp. catnip, powder

- 2 tbsps. elderberries, dried and chopped

- 1 tbsp. rose hips, ground

- Organic chocolate chips or raisins

- Unsweetened grated coconut

Instructions:

1. Combine all the ingredients except the coconut. Mix well with your hands.

2. You will have very firm and pasty candies.

3. Shape balls the size of a nickel with your hands. Roll in the grated coconut. Store the remedy in your refrigerator.

4. I recommend that this candy be consumed 3-4 times a day. Below you will find my dosage chart on how much to give to children of different ages.

Child's Age	Dosage
3-5 years old	½ of one ball each dosage (3 to 4 times a day)
6-11 years old	1 whole ball for a dosage (3 to 4 times a day)
12 years old and above	2 balls for each dosage (3 to 4 times a day)

Make sure they don't try to eat more, as they are very tasty; there is no need for a higher dose.

Constipation

Sometimes children are constipated. This is especially common if they are going through a "difficult" eating phase and are not eating a balanced diet.

Now is a great time to talk to them about the importance of getting their bowels working properly.

Try the following herb candy recipe for relief.

Go Balls

Ingredients:

- 1/4 cup dates (you can also substitute apricots or prunes)

- 1/2 cup hot prune juice

- 1/4 cup almond butter

- 1/8 cup finely ground flax seeds

- 1/8 cup oatmeal.

Instructions:

1. Soak the dates in the prune juice for 15 minutes. Drain the juice and reserve the juice. Place the dates, almond butter, flax seeds, and half of the oatmeal in a food processor. Process until a firm dough form.

2. Add remaining oats or juice as needed to get a very firm consistency using a food processor and then your hands. Shape balls the size of a nickel with your hands.

3. Store the remedy in your refrigerator. Have your child eat this candy 1-2 times a day. Here is a dosage chart to make it easy to remember.

Child's Age	Dosage
3-5 years old	1 ball each dosage (1 to 2 times a day)
6-11 years old	2 balls each dosage (1 to 2 times a day)
12 years old and above	3+ balls for each dosage (1 to 2 times a day)

Roll the balls in ground nuts if your child likes them, as nuts add fiber as well.

Bites, Stings, and Rashes

Insects seem to enjoy the taste of tender skin and warm blood in children. And have you noticed that if there is poison oak, poison ivy, or poison sumac, kids are sure to touch it?

Wash the affected area thoroughly with soap and cold water. Keep the following paste on hand to relieve itching and swelling. The paste speeds up the drying of oozing rashes.

Anti-Itch healing clay

Ingredients:

- 2 tbsp. peppermint leaf (you can substitute 5 drops of peppermint essential oil or 20 drops of tea tree oil)

- 1 cup cosmetic clay (any type will do, but kids love colorful types orange or green)

- 1/3 cup witch hazel extract

- 1/2 cup boiling water

Instructions:

1. Make a very strong tea by covering the peppermint leaf with boiling water.

2. Let stand, covered, for 20 minutes.

3. Once cool, strain the herbs from the liquid. Firmly press the herbs against a colander to get all the healing properties of the mint. Discard the herbs. Reserve the tea.

4. Place the clay in a container with a tight-fitting lid. Pour the witch hazel and herbal tea into the clay, stirring constantly. Add liquid until you get a thick paste.

5. Apply the cover. Carefully label the container, indicating that it is for external use only.

6. If your kids are older and there's no chance they'll eat the dough; keep it in the fridge for freshness. Otherwise, keep it out of reach at room temperature.

7. Apply topically to clean skin whenever insect bites or rashes occur. (It also works on hemorrhoids.) Wash when dry or as desired.

Chapter 4. Modern Herbal Medicine

I cold is a regular occurrence year-round and has been experienced by humanity over, several centuries there are countless number of remedies which have been used and proven without a doubt of their efficacy. tiscommonforpeopletosuggestsomesortofherbal remedy or other if they find you sneezing with watery eyes and stuffy nose. Since the common

While chicken soup, hot steamy vapors, and garlic feature in almost all-herbal common cold remedies, there are some rare remedies that you would not have had the opportunity to come across or try. Here are some very rare but effective herbal remedies for the common cold.

- Eucalyptus oil – This remedy can be taken in the form of few drops in your bath or shower stall for inhalation and easy remedy. For worse cases, an intense treatment method is needed. This involves using about 5 drops of the oil in boiling water and inhaling the vapors arising out of it while being covered by a blanket to trap steam inside. This should be done for a minimum of five to ten minutes and twice a day to clear nasal passages.

- Drinking rose hip flavored tea gives you vitamin C and further prevents the cold from infecting you.

- Apple cider, lemons, and oranges are rich in vitamin C and are best for cold remedies

- The fresh root of ginger helps in avoiding chills

- Onion and garlic added to chicken soup forms an excellent cold fighter food. The antibacterial and antiviral effect of these foods treats cold and prevents it from occurring again

- Spicy foods including chili helps in clearing sinus

- Horseradish is an excellent cold remedy. Eating horseradish sandwich on a daily basis helps in building a strong immunity against the common cold

- Prunes are exceptional cold remedies. Since they are rich in iron, fiber, phosphorus, calcium, vitamins A and B, they help in effective treatment and prevention of the common cold.

- Drinking water in which a whole onion has been boiled also helps.

Powerful Echinacea

This herb helps in developing immunity to the common cold and further reduces the symptoms of the cold and their duration by many days. It helps in stimulating the T-cells important for immunity. When combined with other cold remedies, this herb is excellent for treating the common cold.

The herb is best for preventing all types of infections occurring in the respiratory tract. The incidence and duration of the common cold have been found to decrease drastically when this herb is used. There are two main types of herb preparation used, namely using the above-ground parts of the herb or alcoholic extracts from the root portion. Echinacea tea is also an effective cold remedy.

Andrographis (Andrographis Paniculata)

This safe and effective cold remedy can relieve you of cold symptoms in uncomplicated infections of the upper respiratory tract. The herb has been proved beyond doubt in its effect on reducing the severity of symptoms in common cold and their duration.

Elderberry

This is actually herbal tea made of peppermint and elderflower. Immunity is enhanced largely, and the herb helps in fighting all types of respiratory viruses and influenza. Rapid recovery from the common cold is possible with the extract made from elderberry herb. You can also make the elderberry syrup on your own, which makes it safe and free of chemicals that are often added to store-bought products.

Ginseng and Eleuthero

Ginseng is of various types, and all varieties have been proven to be effective in fighting viruses attacking the respiratory tract. These herbs are especially effective on elderly people. The herb has been used for many years as a remedy for cold.

Licorice Root

Licorice root has several favorable properties, including:

- Antispasmodic—relieves tight coughs

- Demulcent—soothes sore throat

- Anti-inflammatory—reduces the inflamed membrane lining of nose and throat

- Expectorant—helps in expelling mucus in the tract.

The root of licorice is sweet, and when added to other herbal blends, it tastes good. Drinking tea containing licorice root has been recommended to relieve throat pain. The tea has other ingredients, including marshmallow root, elm bark, throat coat, cinnamon bark, orange peel, fenner fruit, and bark of wild cherry tree.

But excess of licorice can lead to kidneys retaining sodium and water while potassium is lost. Limiting the licorice use to about four weeks will prevent unwanted side effects. And it should not be taken in case of pregnancy, low potassium level in blood, with potassium reducing diuretic or in patients with high blood pressure.

Linden Flower

The fever you get with the common cold can be reduced by taking tea made of linden flower. The flower helps in the stimulation of hypothalamus, which is the temperature control region of the body. The tea also induces dilatation of blood vessels resulting in sweating, which brings down the body temperature.

The flower is available as a dried herb. The herb should be steeped in hot water for around 15 minutes. Three or four cups of this tea per day help in reducing high temperature.

A bath in tepid water along with drinking the linden tea helps in keeping your temperature normal.

Toddy

Toddy mixed with lemon juice helps in shortening the duration of cold and in addition, its severity. Honey added to the mix serves to reduce throat ache and boost immunity. The vapors heal the sinuses and open them up, resulting in better relief from the symptoms.

Dark Chocolate

The theobromine in chocolate is far more effective when compared to codeine in suppressing cough. And it does not produce any side effects present in codeine like constipation and drowsiness. One or two squares of chocolate are sufficient to produce the suppressive effect.

Yin Chiao

This is a remedy used in Chinese traditional medicine. It has a blend of herbs, flowers, and roots of forsythia fruit, honeysuckle flower, phragmites rhizome, mint leaf, licorice root, burdock seed, and calcium. The mixture helps in reducing the cold duration effectively. This remedy has been used by the ancient Chinese civilizations to maintain body balance during changing seasons. This over the counter herbal remedy is great for the common cold.

The herbal remedy has immunity-boosting ingredients and antiviral effects, and when taken for three days, it reduces symptoms largely. Sore throat, headache, and nasal congestion are relieved.

Spirulina

Spirulina, a sea algae variety, has good health-promoting ingredients. It is full of antioxidants and rich in selenium and iron. Immunity is greatly enhanced when spirulina is added in tablet or capsule form to the daily diet.

Raw Onions

Onions help in two ways. They are antimicrobial and have sulfur that increases immunity and detoxifies the body.

Munching raw onions or cooking it with vegetables or chicken also helps. But the effect is more when it is eaten in raw form.

Coconut Water

Hydrating the body is vital, especially when affected by the common cold, as you will be losing lots of fluids. Proper hydration can occur only when you get the needed electrolyte. Coconut water is rich in electrolytes and is great for hydration. Bananas, salt, and electrolyte replacing sports drinks also are effective in restoring the electrolyte reserves.

Diet, Exercise, and Rest

While herbal remedies work wonders on your body, you can increase their effect further with some routine lifestyle changes, including:

- Avoid ice cream, popsicles, candies, adding sugar in tea, and any food rich in sugar. It will prolong the cold and make it worse.

  Sugar-free sweeteners or just avoiding sugar altogether also helps.

- When you eat a heavy diet, more time is spent by your body in digesting the food, and the immune system is not focused on. A light diet of soups, fresh veggies, and fruits are easy to digest and boost immunity. Chicken soup, as mentioned before, is great for enhancing immunity and reducing lung inflammation. Onion, yogurt, seaweed, and green tea also help.

- Exercise regularly and in moderation.

- Get adequate rest. When affected by a cold, the body requires more time to deal with the germs and recover. The duration is also reduced when you rest.

- Herbs, including astragalus and olive leaf, also offer ample protection from cold.

- Eating a well-balanced diet is the basic remedial treatment you can do for a cold. A healthy diet predisposes to strong immunity and good health. When you combine herbal remedies with the right diet, rest, and some exercise, you will find your body returning to its normal balance in a short time.

Chapter 5. Plants Used in Herbalism

Detoxification or cleansings depend on the types of fasting that you desire, and trust me, it will do you better if you consume some of the cleansing herbs during your fasting period. However, if you decide to do the water fasting for a week, then throughout that week, you should consume only water and the cleansing herbs in a tea and nothing else should be consumed.

Cascara Sagrada

It is a shrub plant that most people only know it as a "dietary supplement" and was allowed to be sold in the pharmacies as over the counter drugs. However, in 2002, the FDA declares that it doesn't meet the standards to be sold as over-the-counter drugs (OTC) or prescription drugs. Before then, the dietary supplement or the bark of Cascara Sagrada was used as a purgative for constipation. One sweet thing about this shrub is the fact that it is a bitter less extract that can also be used as a flavoring agent.

Rhubarb Root

It is the root and underground stem (that is, rhizome) of the Rhubarb plant. This plant's root has been used by the traditional Chinese people as a medication for the treatment of digestive tract disorder, which includes; stomach pain, constipation, menstrual cramps (dysmenorrhea), diarrhea, swelling of the pancreas, etc. This plant's stems are also used as a flavoring agent and mostly used to make a pie and serve as great recipes. Because of the chemicals that Rhubarb root contains such as fiber, researches have it that it a potent laxative has the potency to reduce swelling, treat cold sores and improves the tone and health of the digestive tract, cleans heavy metal and harmful bacteria, improve the general movement of the intestines and also, reduce cholesterol levels.

Prodigiosa

It is also known as 'Brickellia Grandiflora herb.' It is a flowering plant/shrub from the daisy family and native to Mexico and California. These plant/shrubs have been using by the Mexican as a tea for the treatment of; diarrhea, diabetes, and stomach pain. Research carried on Prodigiosa shows that the plant is an antioxidant; it contains chemical compounds that aid in stimulating the pancreatic gland to secret and reduces or lowers blood sugar level, aid the digestion of fat in the gallbladder, and also, improves the healthiness of the stomach digestive system.

Burdock Root

It is the root of a plant called Burdock that can be found all over the world. Virtually everything about Burdock is important as its root is used as food

and medicine, and its leaf and seed are used for medicinal purposes. A lot of people believe that consuming burdock orally helps to increase the flow of urine, eradicate germs, purify blood, prevent and treat cancer, joint pain, cold, diabetes, anorexia, fever, bladder infections, syphilis, stomach, and intestinal complaints. This plant does not stop there as it also helps in treating and preventing of skin diseases such as; acne and psoriasis. Burdock also helps in boosting of sex drive (libido), lowering of high blood pressure, and cleansing of the liver and lymphatic system.

Dandelion

It is a flowering plant also known as "*Taraxacum officinale*" it is native to Europe. It is commonly found in the mild climates of the northern hemisphere. These flowering plants have been in use for centuries before now for the treatment of swelling (inflammation) of the pancreas, cancer, tonsils (tonsillitis), acne, bladder or urethra, digestive, and liver disorders. Because of the vitamin (A, B, C, E, and K), mineral (iron, potassium, magnesium, and calcium) and other compounds (Polyphenols, Chicoric and Chlorogenic acid) that Dandelion contains, research has it that it has the potency to detoxify gallbladder, kidney and purifies the blood. It also dissolves kidney stones, treats and prevents diabetes, and relieves liver and urinary disorders. It also contains chemicals that may increase urine production, which helps in cleansing the urinary tract and prevent crystals from forming in the urine.

Elderberry

It is also known as European elderberry or black elder, or Sambucus nigra. It is a flowering plant that belongs to Adoxaceae family and the native to Europe. These flowering plants are common in Europe and many other parts of the world. This plant can grow as long as 9 meters. That is 30feet tall and has a lot of clusters (white or cream-colored flowers), which are known as elderflowers. The leaves of elderberry have been used for many years for the treatment of pain, inflammation, swelling, and to stimulate urine production, and to induce sweat. The bark is not left behind as it was also used as a laxative, diuretic, and to induce vomiting.

Guaco

It is a climbing plant that is also known as Guace or Vedolin or Cepu or Bejuco de finca or Liane Francois or Cipo caatinga and other names. This climbing plant is rich with various minerals and compounds. It is from the family of Asteraceae and species of cordifolia. Its leaf is very medicinal and nutritional.

Mullein

It is a flavorful beverage plant that is also known as 'Aaron's rod, Candlewick, American mullein, Adam's flannel, Denseflower mullein, Candleflower, European or orange mullein, etc. this flavorful beverage plant has been used for centuries before now for the treatment of diverse sicknesses, which include; asthma, tuberculosis, pneumonia, chills flu, gastrointestinal bleeding, colds, chronic coughs, and others.

Natural Herbal Tea

According to Alfredo Brownman, or recognized by many as Dr. Sebi, a known herbalist from Honduras, it is important to maintain a "consistent use of natural botanical remedies' and doing so will cleanse and detoxify the body.

While using herbs and natural remedies is an important step in your journey to greater health, you must also remember to make the right adjustments to your eating habits by following the recommended foods list.

We have seen that a plant-based nutrition is fundamental for a healthy diet. But when we talk about plants, we can't consider only fruits and vegetables, in fact, there is also an incredible variety of herbs with a powerful alkaline effect. We need to understand how important they could be for our health: they have a real healing effect that prevents and reverse many diseases.

Herbal medicine is a very ancient practice. It consists of a series of healing techniques based on plants; also, the official modern medicine is aware of the extraordinary properties of many plants and uses them for many common drugs.

We can assume most of their macronutrients in a totally natural way simply through infusions, so we can't neglect them in our alkaline diet. I want to mention a very famous plant: chamomile. Many people use it to relax or sleep, but very few people know its important alkaline effect: when you're stressed or worried, your body increases the production of acid, so a chamomile tea, thanks to its relaxing effect, helps your body to balance its pH value.

Moreover, chamomile fights arachidonic acid, and the result is an important anti-inflammatory effect.

Alfalfa

Also called Lucerne, it is a less know herb with an incredibly high level of nutrients. Its name means "Father of All Foods," in fact, it contains a wide variety of vitamins, minerals, protein, and essential amino acids. Beyond its alkalizing effect, it allows you to reset your metabolism and stay away from different common diseases. More in details, it can:

- Lower the cholesterol level

- Increase immune system functionality

- Clean the blood

- Support digestion

- Alleviate allergies

- Relieve all forms of arthritis

- Relieve headaches and migraines

You should drink alfalfa tea daily, mixing it with another flavored tea if you prefer, since alfalfa is very mild in flavor. Or you could take this herb in capsule form. Whatever you decide, remember that this herb should never be missing; it is one of the biggest secrets for an incredibly healthy life!

Dandelion is another alkaline herb that you can eat as a tea or also as a salad. It is an effective aid against kidney stones, it promotes weight loss, and it contains potent Antioxidants. Dandelion is very rich in vitamin C and folic acid, which are susceptible to heat: for this reason, I suggest you consume this herb as a fresh vegetable, preparing delicious salads with other vegetables. Dandelion is, of course, very cheap, you can easily collect it in the fields or cultivate it in your garden, so you should seriously consider adding this herb to your daily healthy diet.

Red Clover

A particular and almost unknown medicinal herb tea is the one based on red clover. It contains isoflavones, natural phytoestrogens with high antioxidant effects, used for cancer prevention, indigestion, asthma, and bronchitis. Red clover is particularly suitable for women because it promotes female reproductive health, and it may reduce the risk of breast cancer.

There are many herbs that are totally undervalued: usually, people think that their only purpose is to add flavor to our dishes, but they add much more than that. I think, for example, of parsley, basil, cilantro, oregano, sage, and thyme.

Parsley

Parsley is an herb. The leaf, seed, and root are used to make **medicine**. Some people take it by mouth for kidney stones, gastrointestinal disorders, constipation, diabetes, cough, asthma, and high blood pressure.

Nobody knows that parsley contains more vitamin C than oranges! Similarly, it has a very high percentage of vitamin K and a lot of iron.

Basil

It releases into our body high quantities of eugenol, a powerful anti-inflammatory, while oregano is one of the best sources of the free-radical fighters.

Among the other alkaline herbs that we can use to prepare excellent infusions, we can mention lime, sarsaparilla, verbena, sage, and laurel.

Laurel

It is a valid ally against respiratory diseases like flu, bronchitis, cough, and pharyngitis. Moreover, it has positive effects for the treatment of vascular problems and arteriosclerosis. You should also consider buying essential oil, which has antibacterial and antitussive properties.

Chapter 6. Herbal Remedies for Common Ailments

veryday ailments can be easy to treat with basic recipes, simple kitchen tools, and a well-stocked pharmacy of herbs. Whether you have been stung by a Ebee while tending your tomatoes or hit by a flying baseball at your child's Little League game, you'll find a long list of useful remedies here.

Abscess

Painful and hot to the touch, an abscess is an inflamed or infected area filled with pus. The larger an abscess grows, the more painful it becomes. You should seek medical attention if herbal remedies don't help since the infection inside a large abscess can spread to surrounding tissue and into the bloodstream.

Fresh Yarrow Poultice

Makes 1 poultice.

Yarrow contains anti-inflammatory and antibacterial compounds. It works by disinfecting the abscess, easing swelling, and promoting faster healing.

Ingredients:

- 1 tablespoon finely chopped fresh yarrow leaves

Instructions:

1. Apply the chopped leaves to the abscess, then cover with a soft cloth. Leave the poultice in place for 10 to 15 minutes.

2. Repeat two or three times per day until the abscess is healed.

Precautions: Do not use during pregnancy. Yarrow can cause skin reactions in people who are allergic to plants in the Asteraceae family.

Echinacea and Goldenseal Tincture

Makes about 2 cups.

Echinacea and goldenseal offer strong antibacterial benefits, plus they boost your natural immune response. Make this tincture ahead of time, so you have it on hand when you need it. Stored in a cool, dark place, it will last for up to 7 years. Use it any time you have an infection.

Ingredients:

- 5 ounces dried echinacea root, finely chopped

- 3 ounces dried goldenseal root, finely chopped

- 2 cups unflavored 80-proof vodka.

Instructions:

1. In a sterilized pint jar, combine the echinacea and goldenseal. Add the vodka, filling the jar to the very top, and covering the herbs completely.

2. Cap the jar tightly and shake it up. Store it in a cool, dark cabinet and shake it several times per week for 6 to 8 weeks. If any of the alcohol evaporates, add more vodka so that the jar is again full to the top.

3. Dampen a piece of cheesecloth and drape it over the mouth of a funnel. Pour the tincture through the funnel into another sterilized pint jar. Squeeze the liquid from the roots, wringing the cheesecloth until no more liquid comes out. Discard the roots and transfer the finished tincture to dark-colored glass bottles.

4. To treat an abscess, take 10 drops orally two or three times a day for 7 to 10 days.

Precautions: Do not use during pregnancy. Use caution if you have diabetes, as goldenseal can sometimes lower blood sugar.

Acne

Red and swollen, infested sebaceous glands produce aching pimples. Though this ailment typically affects teens, adults can grow it, too. Whether the acne affects only your face or has spread to your chest, back, or other body parts, herbal remedies help you look and feel better.

Calendula Toner

Makes about ½ cup.

With calming calendula that addresses swelling, this simple toner also comprises witch hazel, which goals bacteria whereas unstiffening your skin.

When kept back in a cool, dark place, this toner stays fresh for at least a year.

Ingredients:

- 2 tablespoons calendula oil

- ⅓ cup witch hazel

Instructions:

1. In a dark-colored glass bottle, combine the ingredients and shake gently.

2. With a cotton cosmetic pad, apply 5 or 6 drops to your freshly washed face or other areas of concern. Use a little more or less as needed.

3. Repeat twice per day while acne persists. Store the bottle in the refrigerator if you think you'd like a cooling sensation.

Agrimony-Chamomile Gel

Makes about ⅔ cup.

Agrimony and chamomile, combined with aloe vera gel, soothe redness and ease inflammation. Store the gel in the refrigerator. When kept in an airtight container, it will remain fresh for up to 2 weeks.

Ingredients:

- 2 teaspoons dried agrimony

- 2 teaspoons dried chamomile

- ½ cup water

- ¼ cup aloe vera gel.

Instructions:

1. In a saucepan, combine the agrimony and chamomile with the water. Bring the mix to a boil over high heat, then lessen the heat to low. Boil the mixture until it reduces by half, then remove it from the heat and allow it to cool completely.

2. Dampen a piece of cheesecloth and drape it over the mouth of a funnel. Pour the mixture through the funnel into a glass bowl. Squeeze the liquid from the herbs, wringing the cheesecloth until no more liquid comes out.

3. Add the aloe vera gel to the liquid and use a whisk to blend. Transfer the finished gel to a sterilized glass jar. Cap the jar tightly and store it in the refrigerator.

4. With a cotton cosmetic pad, apply a thin layer to all affected areas twice a day.

Precautions: Omit the chamomile if you take prescription blood thinners or are allergic to plants in the ragweed family.

Allergies

Allergies are abnormal immune responses to a common substance such as cat dander, pollen, or dust. Allergens are found in food, drinks, and the environment, so it's often difficult to avoid them completely. Whereas conventional treatments suppress your body's immune response to allergens that affect you, herbal remedies are far gentler.

Feverfew-Peppermint Tincture

Makes about 2 cups.

Feverfew and peppermint open up the airways during an allergy attack. If you must stay away from feverfew, make this tincture with peppermint alone.

The tincture will keep for up to 7 years in a cool, dark place.

Ingredients:

- 2 ounces dried feverfew

- 6 ounces dried peppermint

- 2 cups unflavored 80-proof vodka

Instructions:

1. In a sterilized pint jar, combine the feverfew and peppermint. Add the vodka, filling the jar to the very top.

2. Cap the jar tightly and shake it up. Store it in a cool, dark cabinet and shake it several times per week for 6 to 8 weeks.

3. Dampen a piece of cheesecloth and drape it over the mouth of a funnel. Pour the tincture through the funnel into another sterilized pint jar. Wring the liquid from the herbs. Discard the spent herbs and transfer the finished tincture to dark-colored glass bottles.

4. Take 5 drops orally whenever allergy symptoms flare-up. If the taste is too strong for you, you can mix it into a glass of water or juice and drink it.

Precautions: Do not use feverfew if you are allergic to ragweed. Do not use feverfew during pregnancy.

Garlic-Ginkgo Syrup

Makes about 2 cups.

Ginkgo biloba is a natural antihistamine that contains more than a dozen anti-inflammatory constituents, while garlic bolsters your immune system. Use local honey if possible, as it can help build resistance to allergens that are found in your area. This syrup will stay fresh for up to 6 months when refrigerated.

Ingredients:

- 2 ounces fresh or freeze-dried garlic, chopped

- 2 ounces ginkgo biloba, crushed or chopped

- 2 cups water

- 1 cup local honey.

Instructions:

1. In a saucepan, combine the garlic and ginkgo biloba with the water. Bring the liquid to a simmer over low heat, cover partially with a lid, and reduce the liquid by half.

2. Transfer the contents of the saucepan to a glass measuring cup, then dispense the mixture over a dampened part of cloth back into the pot, sopping the cheesecloth up until no more fluid comes out.

3. Put the honey and warm the mixture over low heat, constantly stirring and stopping when the temperature reaches 105°F to 110°F.

4. Pour the syrup into a sterilized jar or bottle and store it in the refrigerator.

5. Take 1 tablespoon orally three times per day until your allergy symptoms subside.

Precautions: Do not use if you are consuming a monoamine oxidase inhibitor (MAOI) to address depression. Ginkgo biloba improves the result of blood thinners, so dialog with your doctor before use. Children under age 12 should take 1 teaspoon three times per day.

Asthma

This chronic ailment involves inflamed airways throughout the lungs, along with constricted bronchial tubes. Asthma attacks can be very frightening, so some people also experience panic attacks when breathing becomes difficult.

Ginkgo-Thyme Tea

Makes 1 cup

Ginkgo biloba and thyme help open your airways and relax the muscles in your chest so that you can breathe easier. If you dislike the flavor of this tea, you can add a teaspoon of honey or dried peppermint to the blend to improve its taste.

Ingredients:

- 1 cup boiling water

- 1 teaspoon dried ginkgo biloba

- 1 teaspoon dried thyme.

Instructions:

1. Pour the boiling water into a large mug. Put the dried herbs, cover the mug, and let the tea to sheer for 10 minutes.

2. Relax, then consume the tea gradually while breathing in the steam. Do it again four times in a day.

Safety measures: Do not drink this tea if you are in a monoamine oxidase inhibitor (MAOI) prescription for depression. Ginkgo biloba increases the consequence of blood thinners, so talk to your doctor before use.

Athlete's Foot

This scratchy, occasionally aching infection is produced by a fungus that blooms in humid, warm, dark places. Ensure to cure it before it gets under your toenails, where it will cause discoloration and disfigurement that are very difficult to eradicate.

Fresh Garlic Poultice

Makes 1 treatment

Garlic is a very strong antifungal agent that kills athlete's foot. Raw honey helps bind the garlic to your feet while providing additional antifungal activity. While it's possible to make a double or triple batch of this remedy and use it over the course of 2 to 3 days, you may achieve faster healing by making a fresh batch for each individual treatment.

Ingredients:

- 1 garlic clove, pressed

- 1 teaspoon raw honey.

Instructions:

1. In a small bowl, combine the garlic and honey. With a cotton cosmetic pad, apply the blend to the affected area.

2. Put on a pair of clean socks and relax with your feet up, leaving the poultice in place for 15 minutes to an hour. Wash and dry your feet afterward. Repeat the treatment once or twice per day, and follow up with an application of Goldenseal Ointment (HERE). Continue for 3 days after symptoms disappear.

Precautions: Garlic may cause a skin rash in sensitive individuals.

Goldenseal Ointment

Makes about 1 cup.

Goldenseal is a potent antimicrobial agent that helps put a stop to athlete's foot. You can use this ointment on its own or speed healing by using it in concert with a Fresh Garlic Poultice (<u>HERE</u>). It will stay fresh for up to a year when stored in a cool, dark place.

Ingredients:

- 1 cup light olive oil

- 2 ounces dried goldenseal root, chopped

- 1-ounce beeswax

Instructions:

1. In a slow cooker, combine the olive oil and goldenseal. Select the lowest heat setting, cover the slow cooker, and allow the roots too steep in the oil for 3 to 5 hours. Turn off the heat and allow the infused oil to cool.

2. Bring an inch or so of water to a simmer in the base of a double boiler. Reduce the heat to low.

3. Drape a piece of cheesecloth over the upper half of the double boiler. Pour in the infused oil, then wring and twist the cheesecloth until no more oil comes out. Discard the cheesecloth and spent herbs.

4. Add the beeswax to the infused oil and place the double boiler on the base. Gently warm over low heat. When the beeswax melts completely, remove the pan from the heat. Quickly pour the mixture into clean, dry jars or tins and allow it to cool completely before capping.

5. With a cotton cosmetic pad, apply ¼ teaspoon to each affected area. Use a little more or less as needed, and repeat up to three times per day, with the final application being before bed. Wear a pair of clean socks over the ointment to prevent slipping.

Precautions: Do not use if you are pregnant or breastfeeding. Do not use if you have high blood pressure.

Chapter 7. Herbs for Beauty and Vitality

Alternative medicine isn't the only thing people are looking into today for overall health. Herbs that are used for natural care of the hair, body, and skin are also quite popular. Herbs that help with energy, memory, and overall vitality are quite popular as well.

So many people today are concerned with the synthetic chemicals that are being used in beauty products such as lotions, make-up, and soaps because of allergic reactions and toxins that may be released into the body. Our bodies are bombarded daily with environmental pollutants like carbon emissions, heavy metals, and exhaust fumes that can harm the cells in the body.

If you really take a long look at research and information regarding the ingredients in some make-up and other grooming products, you may be surprised at what you find. For example, musk is a dried secretion from the genitals of otters, beavers, musk deer, and civet cats. However, most musk's now are synthetic. Musk has been linked to gynecological problems because of the way estrogen reacts with it. There are some all-natural musky alternatives if you enjoy the smell. They come from pungent plants. Collagen and elastin are derived from the connective tissue of animals which is found in many types of facial moisturizers and wrinkle treatments. Another example is Hyaluronic Acid, which is taken from rooster combs. It has been deemed safe, and it is recommended to hydrate and plump the skin. Hyaluronic acid can be found in many creams, skin masks, and lipsticks that promote moisture and plumping. If you are looking to remove animal products from all aspects of your life, you may want to look into herbal alternatives to animal products. There are all-natural pigments and dyes available as well.

There are plenty of herbs that have been used for centuries to help keep the body, mind, and spirit healthy. Many of the herbs are still used today. Some people look for products that are specifically made with organic ingredients because of their raw nature. In many cases, it is simply easier to purchase your own herbs and make your own products at home. In some cases, it is much cheaper, and you know exactly where the things that you are putting in your body are coming from.

Below, we will list 10 of the best herbal remedies that can be used to improve your health through the skin and hair care, mood improvement, memory improvement, and improve your energy. These examples are also a good place to start if you wish to start getting chemicals out of your home and replacing them with all-natural solutions.

Turmeric

Turmeric is a super spice. It not only gives an incredible flavor to curry and other Indian foods; it also has many health benefits. Its flavor is very potent and quite spicy. It is also full of powerful antioxidants and is known to be anti-inflammatory. It is a shrub that grows in Asia and Western India and has been used in Ayurveda and Chinese medicine for centuries.

Upon its discovery, it was used mainly as a spice and a dye because of its bright yellow color. The bright yellow color comes from curcumin, a compound that is found in turmeric. It has also been used in religious ceremonies and at festivals in India as a dye for robes, saris, and it is used to decorate the body as ornamentation.

Turmeric is so sacred that it is used in wedding rituals and ceremonies in India, Pakistan, and Bangladesh. The spice is used for bridal beautification ceremonies. It helps to cleanse the body and give the skin a radiant, golden glow.

Turmeric is a great spice to use for skincare. It has many benefits. Turmeric can treat blemishes and blackheads on the skin, hyper-pigmentation, and dark spots. It has also been used as a treatment for psoriasis and eczema. It helps to heal dry skin and prevents it from returning.

Turmeric also slows the aging process. It is used to keep the skin soft and supple by improving its elasticity and elevating wrinkles. Turmeric is also being used in sunscreen products to give a person that radiant glow and protect against drying of the skin. East Indian women use it daily as a facial wash and exfoliant.

Look for Kasturi turmeric, as regular turmeric can stain the skin temporarily. It can only be used externally and isn't the same spice that is used for cooking. It is generally mixed with Gram flour (chickpea, garbanzo bean flour) and milk. The flour helps exfoliate while the milk removes dead skin cells.

There are several different recipes for homemade exfoliants, cleansers, and skin brighteners;

To reduce wrinkles, mix turmeric with milk. To brighten the skin, simply add rice powder with milk and tomato juice and apply the paste to the face and neck. You can also exfoliate by adding rice flour, yogurt or soy milk, and turmeric to make a paste that can be placed upon the skin.

Turmeric is also an excellent facial hair reducer. Mix the turmeric with chickpea flour and leave it on the face for about 15 minutes. You should see results in about a month.

Turmeric can be added to a bit of your favorite moisturizer, night cream, or acne treatment if you don't want to make your own recipe. Simply apply to the face and wash it off in about 15 minutes.

Turmeric relieves oily skin because it reduces the production of sebum, or naturally occurring skin oils.

You can also buy turmeric exfoliating creams and masks online and at local health food stores. One good example is *Juara's Turmeric Antioxidant Radiance Mask*. It can be a bit pricey; however, it can be worth it just to reap the benefits of turmeric.

Schisandra

Schisandra berries are very powerful. The plant is a woody vine that grows primarily in Korea, China, and Russia. The berries are eaten regularly, and they are quite sweet and flavorful. They are often dried, cooked, or eaten raw. They contain adaptogen. Adaptogen is defined as any plant substance that can enhance the body in a nonspecific way and helps the body resist any form of stress. Adaptogens do not cause harm to the body, and they are beneficial to the body by balancing it instead of overstimulating it.

Adaptogens are used as overall wellness supplements. They promote health but don't particularly treat any type of illness.

Schisandra is a well-protected herb in China as it is used by many as a wellness tonic. Schisandra increases your capacity for physical and mental exercise by giving you balanced energy. It stimulates the central nervous system without creating the shaky, nervous side effects that caffeine or some other supplements can cause. It also has a calming effect on the nervous system when the body is faced with mental or physical stress. It can also help protect your body from environmental stress such as pollutants. People who suffer from depression, anxiety, and other mood disorders find Schisandra very helpful.

Athletes are known to take Schisandra as it increases energy and nitric oxide levels. On the other end of the spectrum, it fights fatigue. All of the benefits of Schisandra are seen at the cellular level.

Studies have shown that Schisandra can raise the body's enzyme and glutathione, which helps mental clarity.

It can also keep the liver healthy and functioning properly by filtering out toxins. In China, it is used to help with the treatment of Hepatitis C because of the benefits to the liver.

For men, Schisandra can help with impotence and erectile dysfunction since it helps blood vessels dilate, causing an erection. Blood vessel dilation can also help with other problems such as high blood pressure.

It is great for the skin as well because of its many detoxifying properties and is used for anti-aging and longevity. Schisandra was very popular with the Chinese emperors, and it was used as an anti-aging tonic to help reduce stress and fatigue. The ladies were also quite fond of Schisandra for use on their skin.

Ginseng

Ginseng root has been a part of Chinese and Korean medicine for centuries. North American ginseng was used in Native American medicine as well. There are quite a few types of ginseng that grow all over the world. The strains that are the most sought after are the Asian variety (Panax ginseng) and the American variety (where the root is used). Panax ginseng was used in Traditional Chinese Medicine as an agent to improve circulation and increase the blood supply. It was also used to help people who had been ill to recover quicker from the illness as it helped to improve weakness. Ginseng also stimulates the body.

American ginseng, according to Traditional Chinese Medicine, detoxifies and calms the body.

Both varieties of ginseng plants grow wild. They are also cultivated. You can also grow your own ginseng. Wild ginseng can be either the American or Asian varieties, and it is quite rare because it takes years for the root to reach maturity. Also, the high demand is wiping out the wild population. There are some programs, for example, in Tennessee, Maine, and West Virginia, where the plants are grown in the woods to restore it to its natural habitat.

American and Asian ginseng are adaptogens, just like Schisandra. It has been used as an aphrodisiac and for sexual dysfunction. Both types of ginseng promote libido and sexual performance. The compounds contained in ginseng stimulate the central nervous system and male hormones.

It has also been used to improve mental clarity and energy levels.

Rose Hips

Rose hips are berries that are left behind by a rose bush after the flower has fallen off. Nearly all types of rose bushes will produce rose hips. Rose hips have been used in perfumes and in candies, syrups, and other confections to give them a sweet taste.

The berries are high in vitamin C, and the fatty acids that are contained within them have tissue regenerating properties. Rose water and rose oil has been used in the past to treat eye irritations as well. Rose hips have anti-inflammatory properties and are being tested for use as a pain reliever for arthritis relief.

Witch Hazel

Witch hazel was used by Native Americans for many different purposes. Witch hazel is a great astringent. It is produced from the leaves and bark of the witch hazel shrub that is native to Canada and the United States.

Witch hazel leaves and twigs are steamed to make the astringent. You may have seen witch hazel in many pharmacies. However, the witch hazel that is sold in drug stores can be harsh and may contain alcohol. Essential oils can't be made with witch hazel because there isn't enough oil in the plant. If you want a milder witch hazel, check with your local health food store or online.

Witch hazel has so many uses, especially for skincare and beauty. It can be used for pimples and acne. If you have ever heard of putting hemorrhoid cream under your eyes to reduce bags, it is a tried and true beauty tip. The main ingredient in hemorrhoid creams is witch hazel. The astringent tightens up the skin and reduces sagging. That being said, it also shrinks hemorrhoid tissues externally. It helps reduce itching and will dry up any bleeding.

Chapter 8. Recipes

White Turnip Herbal Soup

S procedure, calm, constant dry skin, and enhance the discharge of sexual hormones. In this recipe, we join it with a white turnip, another herb that assists with clearing the lungs from mucus and cool the body. White turnip is also viable for controlling ceaseless cough and purifying the skin.

Preparation time: 5 mins

Cooking time: 25 mins.

Serves: 4

Ingredients:parklyAsparagus is a popular herb well known for its saturating properties. It is regularly used to reestablish vitality after an illness or a medical

- 1¼ liters (5 cups) of water

- 15 g (½ oz.) of Shiny Asparagus (tian men doing), washed

- 300 g (10 oz.) white turnip, cut into meager cuts

- 1 teaspoon salt, or to taste

- 1 teaspoon newly ground black pepper

- 1 spring onion, minced, to garnish

Preparation:

1. Bring 500 ml (2 cups) of the water to a boil in a saucepan over medium heat. Add the herb and stew revealed until the water has diminished to half, about 20 minutes.

Expel from the heat and strain the stock with a cloth or fine strainer. Save the clear stock and discard the residue.

2. Allow the remaining water to boil in a saucepan, pour in the clear stock, and add the turnip cuts. Diminish the heat to low, spread, and stew for 5 to 8 minutes, until the turnip is delicate.

3. Remove from the heat. Add pepper and salt, then blend well. Serve hot and garnished with spring onion.

Poached Eggs and Mushroom in Clear Broth

This is a tonic soup with high nutritional value. Pine seeds are an excellent supplement for enhancing quality and endurance. Eggs are a rich wellspring of protein and essential fatty acids, and the supplement required for extra quality and stamina. Attempt to purchase the eggs of organically took care of unfenced chickens. These give a far preferable nutritional profile over the ordinary mass-delivered eggs. The chicken stock further improves the nutritional and tonic value of this fortifying soup.

Preparation time: 20 mins + 30 mins to soak

Cooking time: 1 hour 20 mins

Serves: 5

Ingredients:

- 3 liters (12 cups) water

- 15 g (½ oz.) pine seeds (tune zi), flushed and squashed

- 1 tablespoon rice vinegar, weakened with 1 liter (4 cups) water

- 5 eggs 750 g (1½ lbs.) chicken parts, cleaned

- 1 tablespoon rice wine

- ½ teaspoon salt

- ½ teaspoon newly ground black pepper

- 5 large dried shiitake mushrooms, and soaked in boiling water until delicate, stems discarded, caps cut into slight strips

- 1 spring onion, cut.

Preparation:

1. Allow the remaining water to boil in a stockpot over high heat. Add the pine seeds, diminish the heat to low, and stew them for 30 mins, until the water decreases to about two-third. Expel from the heat and strain the stock with a cloth or fine strainer. Save

   the clear stock and discard the leftovers.

2. Bring the weakened rice vinegar to a boil in a saucepan. Diminish the heat to low and keep it stewing. Individually, break the eggs and delicately place them into the pan. Poach the eggs for about one moment; at that point, expel carefully with a slotted spoon, wash in cool water, and put aside on a plate.

3. Bring the pine seed stock to a boil, add the chicken parts, and lessen the heat to low, and boil for 45 minutes. Expel from the heat and strain. Hold the clear stock and discard the bones and parts.

4. Bring the pine seed chicken stock to a boil, season with the wine, salt, and pepper, then add the cut mushroom and spring onion. Lessen the heat to a delicate stew, add the poached eggs, and keep on stewing for 1 more moment. Expel from the heat.
5. Ladle one egg and some mushroom into five individual serving bowls; at that point, ladle the stock over and serve hot. Instead of eggs, you may also prepare this soup with new prawns as the main nutritional ingredient. For additional flavor, sprinkle each serving bowl with some slashed new coriander leaves (cilantro). You may also add a dash of Chinese sesame oil for a nutty flavor and additional tonic value, especially in winter.

Lingzhi Lean Pork Soup

For a considerable length of time, the Chinese recommended Lingzhi, a mushroom kind, as the "lord of herbs" for its excellent impact in improving overall health, enhancing stamina, and advancing life span. It is advanced as an immune system promoter, a blood pressure stabilizer, and an antioxidant. Joined with red dates, Wild Yam, and Wolfberry, this soup is excellent in fortifying and supporting the body. However, one ought not to drink this soup while having a typical cold.

Preparation time: 5 mins

Cooking time: 2 hours 45 mins

Serves: 4-6

Ingredients:

- 2½ liters (10 cups) water

- 19 g (3/5 oz.), flushed and cut

- 19 g (3/5 oz.) Wild Yam, washed

- 5 rutted red dates, washed

- 350 g (12 oz.) lean pork, washed and burned with hot water

- 2 tablespoons Chinese Wolfberry, and washed

- 1 teaspoon salt, or to taste

Preparation:

1. Heat the water to the point of boiling in a stockpot. Add all the ingredients, aside from the salt, and cook over high heat for 10 minutes.

49

2. Diminish the heat to low, and stew revealed for 2½ hours. Season with the salt and expel from the heat. Serve hot.

Brown Rice and Bamboo Shoots Cooked in Dodder Broth

Dodder is a traditional Chinese herbal solution for male barrenness and urinary tract issues. Besides, its property has a sexual tonic; it also reinforces bone and ligament, calms lumbago, and balances the female reproductive system. The small seeds, which have a savory flavor, are boiled straightforwardly with rice, enhancing the taste of this dish and protecting maximum therapeutic power.

Preparation time: 5 mins

Cooking time: 50 mins

Serves: 4

Ingredients:

- 200 g (1 cup) uncooked brown rice, washed in a few changes of water, and drained

- 200 g (7 oz.) new bamboo shoot, stripped and diced

- 625 ml (2½ cups) water

- 10 g (⅓ oz.) Chinese Dodder seeds (tu si zi), flushed and placed in a zest bag

- 2 teaspoons soy sauce

- ½ teaspoon salt, or to taste

- 2 tablespoons rice wine

- 1 teaspoon sugar.

Preparation:

1. In a large saucepan or stockpot, carry all the ingredients to a full boil. Diminish the heat to the low, spread firmly with a top, and stew for about 45 minutes until you tenderly cook the rice and all it has absorbed all the water.

2. Expel from the heat and serve in individual serving bowls.

3. For stronger flavors, various sauces, such as sesame oil, Szechuan pepper-salt powder, bean stew paste, and minced spring onion, may be served along with the dish on the table to suit individual taste.

Fish Ball Spinach Soup

Achyranthes, known as "Bull Knee" in Chinese, is a traditional female tonic that rectifies menstrual disorders. It is also a general liver and kidney tonic for old people, advancing blood circulation, cleansing the bloodstream, and easing pains in the lower back and waist. It also stimulates the energy stream in the meridians. We join this recipe with new handmade fish balls and prawns to balance its therapeutic and nutritional values.

Preparation time: 30 mins

Cooking time: 25 mins

Serves: 4

Ingredients:

- 15 g (½ oz.) Achyranthes Root (niu xi)

- 1 ½ liter (6 cups) water

- 300 g (10 oz.) white fish filets, cleaned, minced

- 1 egg

- 1½ teaspoons lotus root powder or cornstarch, blended in with 4 tablespoons water

- 125 g (4 oz.) new prawns, stripped and deveined

- 125 g (4 oz.) spinach, stemmed, slashed

- 1 teaspoon soy sauce.

- 1 teaspoon salt, or as you desire

- ½ teaspoon newly ground black pepper

Preparation:

1. Bring the herb and ½ litter (2 cups) of the water to a boil in a saucepan. Diminish the heat to low, spread, and stew for about 15 minutes, until the blend decreased to about half. Expel from the heat, strain, and hold the clear stock. Discard the leftovers.
2. Combine the fish, egg, and lotus root powder or cornstarch blend in a bowl and blend well.

3. Allow the remaining water to a boil in a stockpot over high heat. Spoon 1 heaped tablespoon of the fish blend, wet your hands, and shape it into a ball, then drop it gently into the boiling water. When the fish ball is cooked, it will float to the boiling water surface. Evacuate the cooked fish ball with a slotted spoon and transfer to a bowl. Keep on making the fish balls in the same manner with the remaining fish blend.

4. Add the shrimp and spinach to the same pot of boiling water, and season with the soy sauce, salt, and pepper. Pour in the herb stock and return the soup to a boil. Finally, add the cooked fish balls, stew revealed for 2-3 minutes, and expel from the heat.
5. Serve hot in a large soup tureen or individual serving bowls. For example, different vegetables, such as white turnip, bok choy, or new mushrooms, maybe good in addition instead of the spinach. You may incorporate

clams or shellfish with or in place of the shrimp. New hacked coriander leaves (cilantro) may be added as a garnish to give extra flavor.

Miso Fish Soup With Daikon

Wild Yam is a tonic to the spleen's elements, stomach, and lungs, and it also helps regulate hormone production in ladies. Late research has shown that this herb brings down the blood sugar level and may, along these lines, assists with controlling diabetes. It enhances these properties when joined with the minerals and trace components given in this recipe by new fish and seaweed.

Preparation time: 30 mins

Cooking time: 15 mins

Serves: 4

Ingredients:

- 750 ml (3 cups) of water

- 1 piece of kombu seaweed (5 cm/2 in since a long time ago), cut the strips into 3 pieces

- (15 g) Wild Yam (huai shan), soaked in water, at that point mashed into the paste

- 150 g (5 oz.) Diakon radish stripped and destroyed

- 5 tablespoons miso paste

- 300 g (10 oz.) white fish filets (snakehead or grouper), cut the pinch of newly ground black pepper, and sliced the spring onion to garnish.

Preparation:

1. Allow the remaining water to boil in a saucepan. Add the seaweed strips, spread, and stew for about 3 minutes. Add the daikon, Wild Yam, and miso pastes, blend well

and come back to a boil. Diminish the heat to low, spread, and stew for 5 minutes.
2. Increase the gas or stove to medium, add the fish cuts, and cook for about 2 minutes or until cook. Expel from the heat.

3. Sprinkle some black pepper to the soup and garnish with cut spring onion. Scoop into individual serving dishes and serve hot. Instead of kombu, you may also use different seaweed in this soup. If you don't care for Daikon, you may eliminate it without diminishing the soup's therapeutic efficacy. Szechuan peppercorn-salt powder may be used instead of black pepper for extra zing.

Chapter 9. How to Make Herbal Medicine and Infusions

ᴍ aking herbal medicines is easy and fun. With a few simple tools and ingredients, you can transform your herbs into all manner of delicious and effective remedies.

Essential Tools and Equipment:

- *Mason jars.* These are the herbalist's best friend. Because they're made of heat-resistant glass, you can pour boiling water right into them to make tea. They're also handy for making tinctures, storing herbs, and more. Quart- and pint-size jars are the most versatile, though for storing dry herbs, you may want larger jars. Many store-bought foods (sauerkraut, salsa, etc.) come in mason jars—just hand wash or run them through the dishwasher and dry to reuse them.

- *Wire mesh strainers.* For straining tea or pressing out tinctures, you'll want strainers of various sizes. Start with a few single-mug strainers for making one cup of tea at a time, as well as a larger, bowl-size strainer for filtering larger amounts of herb-infused liquids.

- *Cheesecloth.* This is handy not only for straining and squeezing herbs you've infused into the liquid but also for wrapping the herbs in a poultice.

- *Measuring cups and spoons.* Cup, tablespoon, and teaspoon measures are all helpful, as well as some graduated measuring cups with pour spouts, which allow you to measure down to a quarter ounce.

- *Funnels.* A set of small funnels is extremely helpful for getting tinctures and other liquids into bottles with small openings.

- *Bottles.* For storing tinctures long term, amber or blue glass bottles are best. The "Boston round" type is a

- favorite for tinctures and other liquid remedies, but any shape will do. Get in the habit of saving and reusing any colored glass bottles you come across —there are a number of kombucha brands that come in amber glass, for instance.

- One- and two-fluid-ounce bottles are most convenient for dose bottles, while storage bottles are usually 4 to 12 fluid ounces. For storage, use plain bottle caps, but you'll need dropper tops for dose bottles.

- *Labels.* Label your remedies as soon as you make them. Address labels are sufficient for most purposes—even a bit of masking tape will do in a pinch.

- *Blender.* For mixing lotions, breaking down bulky fresh plant matter, and other purposes, a standard kitchen blender will serve just fine.

Nice-to-Have Equipment

These tools make it easier to integrate herbs into your life, especially if you have a busy schedule, but they're not as necessary as those preceding.

- *French press.* This is our favorite tool for making herbal infusions. It allows the herb material to float freely in the water and exposes a lot of surface area for extraction (you just press down to easily dispense filtered tea), and it is simple to clean.

- *Thermos.* When traveling or bringing your tea to work, a good thermos is an asset. There are versions that include a filter built directly into the lid, so you can put the herbs and water directly into the thermos together from the start.

- *Press pot.* This is an insulated pot with a lever you press to dispense. People usually put coffee or strained tea into these, though we've found you can usually get away with putting herbs directly into the pot, pouring in boiling water, and letting it infuse in there. It'll stay hot all day, and you just dispense it by the cup. (Hold a little mesh

•

strainer under the spout to catch any herb bits that pass through the tube.)

•   *Herb grinder.* A simple, small coffee grinder served us well for many years, but if you plan to make a lot of herb powders, you may want a larger, dedicated machine.

Helpful Ingredients

Herbs and water alone will serve for a great many remedies, but some preparations require additional ingredients.

•   *Alcohol.* Tinctures are mixtures of herb extracts and alcohol. We usually use vodka or brandy.

•   *Apple cider vinegar.* Always use this, rather than distilled white vinegar, for herb-infused vinegar, oxymels (a blend of vinegar and honey), and topical applications.

•   *Honey.* Choose local honey whenever possible, unprocessed/unfiltered if you can get it. Beware that some big-brand of honey have been found to be contaminated or even contain high fructose corn syrup. Liquid honey is easiest to use in herbal honey

infusions, while thicker honey can be more manageable for first aid and wound care.

•   *Oils.* You can use olive oil for most purposes, though in some instances, you'll want a lighter oil, such as grapeseed or almond, or a thicker oil such as shea butter or cocoa butter. You can even use animal-derived oils, such as lard, tallow, or lanolin.

•   *Beeswax.* Salves require wax to thicken them. You can buy beeswax in rounds or chunks and cut it down for each use. You can also buy beeswax pellets, which can be easier to work with.

- *Witch hazel extract.* Look for a witch hazel extract made without alcohol, as this is most versatile—especially for first aid or wound care.

- *Rose water.* Traditionally used for skin care, though also as a food ingredient. Rose water from the "ethnic foods" section of the grocery store is just as good as the higher-priced stuff in the health and beauty aisle.

- *Sea salt and Epsom salts.* For baths and soaks as well as nasal sprays and gargles, a bit of salt improves the medicine.

- *Gelatin capsules.* The "oo" size is most frequently used when working with herbal powders to make homemade herb capsules.

Safety Tips

- *Label everything.* If you don't know what you're taking, you can't be sure it's safe. Include details about all the ingredients in the remedy, as well as the date it was made.

- *Start small.* Begin with small test batches and small doses when working with a new remedy. You can always scale up or take more later, but if an herb or preparation doesn't agree with you, it's best to discover that with a small amount.

- *Be cautious with pharmaceuticals.* Herbs and pharmaceutical drugs (including both prescription and over-the-counter medications) can interact in many ways. Sometimes this is beneficial—positive herb-drug interactions may allow someone to reduce the dose of a drug or minimize its side effects—but it is a complicated subject and should be handled very carefully.

We identify the major interactions to watch for in the notes that accompany each remedy, but it's always best to consult with a practicing herbalist familiar with this topic or your health care provider, especially if multiple drugs are taken simultaneously.

Best Practices

Use your senses. Look at the herbs you're working with and your finished product. Check for mold in your jar of infused oil, check for bits of packaging material in your shipment of dried herbs. *Smell and taste* your herbs and remedies to get a sense of their potency, and dose accordingly.

Make only what you need. If you get great results from a particular remedy and you want to have it on hand every day, great—go for it. But no one needs a gallon of nasal spray solution, and it'll go bad before you even get around to using it. Make only those remedies you need, and only as much as you need.

Begin with what's abundant. In this book, we focus on herbs that are highly prevalent in the wild or grown commercially on a large scale. As you branch out into working with other plants, keep your focus on those that are local to you and neither at risk nor endangered. Don't be tricked into thinking a rare, exotic herb will be the only one to solve your problem—it's vanishingly rare for that to be true.

Get the herb to the tissue. Herbs need to be in contact with the affected tissue to help it. We can't always just drink some herbal tea and get good results. Choose a delivery method that helps your herbs get where they need to act.

A few examples: If you're working with a respiratory problem, go with a steam; if you've got something on the skin, apply a soak or poultice; if it's trouble in the lower intestine, swallow some powder, so it's intact when it gets down there.

Infusions

If you think of making tea, you probably picture an infusion. It's the simplest, most fundamental way to work with herbs and is our preferred method in most circumstances. Infusions can be prepared in a variety of ways, but these are the most common:

- *Hot infusion.* Like using a tea bag, a short, hot infusion means pouring boiling water on your herbs, letting them steep for a few minutes, and drinking as soon as tolerably cool. This method is best for herbs with aromatic or volatile constituents, which will evaporate if left to infuse too long.

- *Cold infusion.* This method is used for demulcent, or mucilaginous, herbs, such as marshmallow—those that increase the water's viscosity as they infuse, rendering it first "velvety," then slimy. This only happens in cold water; hot water doesn't release the constituents responsible for this effect.

- *Long infusion.* When trying to extract mineral content from nutritive herbs such as nettle, a long infusion is required. When done in a tightly sealed jar, this method also allows us to combine the quick-release aromatic constituents of one herb with the slow-release mucilage from another, as the initially hot water cools over time.

Administration and Dosage Guidelines

Infusions are generally drunk as they are. It can also aid as an ingredient in alternative remedies (compress, lotion, bath, soak, syrup, and more). Each
permeated herb or formula has its own prescription arrays, but, for most in this book, it is normal to take a quart of infusion every day, occasionally more.

Shelf Life and Storing Rules

Dry herbs mixed for an infusion can be saved for years, given that they are stored in airtight vessels. Once water is placed, infusions are generally only good for 1 or 2 days; if kept refrigerated, this could extend to 3 days. Trust your tongue: If the tea tastes "skunky" or otherwise off, best to make a new batch.

Necessary Tools, Equipment, or Ingredients

- Herbs

- Water

- Teacup, teapot, mason jar, French press, or another container

- Mesh strainer

Preparing Remedies: Step-by-Step Instructions

1. Unless otherwise specified, use 2 to 3 tablespoons of herbs per quart of water. (If making only a single cup of tea, use 1 to 3 teaspoons of herbs.)

2. Combine the herbs with the water and let steep:

  - *Hot infusion.* Pour boiling water over the herbs, cover, and steep for 20 minutes or until cool enough to drink.

  - *Cold infusion.* Pour cold or room-temperature water over the herbs and steep for 4 to 8 hours.

  - *Long infusion.* Pour boiling water over the herbs, cover tightly, and steep for 4 to 8 hours or overnight.

3. Once the herbs have steeped, you may strain the liquid and compost the *marc* (leftover herb material).

Pros

- *Easy to make.* Hot water, herbs, and a container are all you need.

- *Versatile.* Infusions can be employed in a variety of ways, depending on need.

- *Potent.* Each infusion method extracts a broad spectrum of constituents from the herbs, giving a good reflection of their full potential.

- *Hydrating.* Drinking enough water is important for good health; infusions count as water intake.

Chapter 10. Herbal Medicines for Immune System Protection

The Immune System

Functional and metabolic regulation. In human beings, it is the ability to maintain the aforementioned balance while managing the challenges which require mental, physical, and social energy on a daily basis. According to the World Health Organization, health is a state where there is absolute allhaveadesiretostayhealthyandyouthful,andwechaselongevityallourlives.H ealthorbeinghealthyreferstothebody'sbalancebetweenits well-being when it comes to physical, mental, and social areas as well as the absence of any kind of infection, disease, and illness. More recent studies indicate that health involves balance in living organisms in the form of integral and harmonious performance of basic functions, which in turn helps the individual develop normally. The body's ability to defend and fight against diseases is known as immunity. It is also responsible for preventing allergies and enduring autoimmune diseases. A strong and well-functioning immune system means good health.

The most important defense system in the human body is the immune system, which protects the body against various threats and harmful microorganisms, eventually preventing serious illnesses. It works by interacting with different types of cells, organs, and tissues present in the body while maintaining cooperation and regulating the whole system effectively. The immune system is spread over the primary and secondary lymphoid organs, mostly at the mucosa of the lungs and the gastrointestinal tract, and the skin. All immune cells are derived from pluripotent hematopoietic stem cells in the bone marrow. The differentiation process starts with the appearance of myeloid and lymphoid stem cells. The differentiation then occurs in the lymphocytes of the T and B lineages that are located within the bone marrow and the thymus. The result of effective interaction between the components, both natural and adaptive, within the immune system is known as immune response.

Disorders Related to Immune System

An immense amount of interest in the immune system has risen in the last three decades, and it has been recognized as an essential defender of the human body. Moreover, most harmful drugs, chemicals, and pollutants in the environment target the immune system as well. Since immune cells continue to experience differential and get renewed regularly in order to maintain immunity, the entrance of foreign substances in the body can affect the immune system greatly. This may also result in toxic alteration within the immune system.

In the same way, the modulation of the immune system, or immunomodulation, is also an important process of the immune system. It helps to preserve health and prevents diseases and illnesses from entering the body. This concept is receiving well-deserved recognition all around the world since the number of people contracting life-threatening diseases has been increasing. The world is witnessing more and more patients being diagnosed with cancer, in need of transplants, and with AIDS. The number of diseases and infections resistant to available antibiotics has also been rising to a concerning degree. The effectiveness of antibiotics has been decreasing, resulting in people preferring self-medication. Pharmacological actions on some components of the immune response are being considered as an alternative approach to therapy against diseases. The immunologic control of diseases helps to develop immunity as well as prevent undesired immune reactions.

Herbal Medicine to Strengthen the Immune System

Plants are essentially the biosynthetic carriers of phytochemicals. Phytochemicals are the natural compounds found in biologically active plants. Also known as secondary metabolites, these compounds are classified into different classes, including alkaloids, flavonoids, coumarins, glycosides, gums, polysaccharides, phenols, tannins, terpenes, and terpenoids. Secondary metabolites are synthesized by plant cells. They are produced as a response to external stimulants such as infections and climatic and nutritional changes. The phytochemicals in plants are responsible for their protection and the presence of colors, flavors, and aroma. Other than that, they also come with therapeutic effects and some anti-oxidant, anti-diabetic, memory-enhancing, cholesterol-lowering, adaptogen, anti-cancer, and immunomodulatory abilities. For this reason, herbal medicines are very popular, and to add to this, they also contain little to no side effects.

Turmeric

Botanical name: Curcuma longa, Curcuma domestica

Commercial turmeric of commerce is the dried rhizome of the plant and used in traditional medicine, nutraceuticals, and as biopesticide, too. Turmeric is valued mainly for its principal yellow coloring pigment, curcumin. Besides curcumin, other related pigments such as dimethoxy curcumin and bis-dimethoxy curcumin, which also impart the yellow color, are all together called curcuminoids.

Medicinal uses: *Curcuma longa* has been used for thousands of years as a medicine in old-style Indian and traditional medicine for the treatment of a large assortment of illnesses, that includes infectious diseases, inflammation, gastric, hepatic, and blood disorders.

The biological activity of turmeric is anti-inflammatory, spasmolytic, antihepatotoxic, antibacterial, hypercholesteremic, antimicrobial, antiviral, cytotoxic, choleretic, hypersensitive, antirheumatic, and antidiabetic. Turmeric is also famous for its anti-cancer properties. Curcumin has been used as a remedy for the prevention and treatment of many organ and tissue disorders, most of which are associated with inflammation and oxidative stress, e.g., Alzheimer's disease and Parkinson's disease.

Cinnamon

Botanical name: Cinnamomum verum

Cinnamon is an age-old spice. Cinnamon is endemic to Sri Lanka, which is the major producer and exporter of bark oil and leaf oil. Seychelles,

Madagascar, and India also produce cinnamon bark, though in small quantities. The bark oil consists of cinnamaldehyde, eugenol, and eugenol acetate as major therapeutic ingredients. Bark oil is a pale yellow with a strong, warm, sweet, spicy, tenacious odor and a sweet and pungent taste.

Medicinal uses: Cinnamon has been used therapeutically for thousands of years to match toothache, clean up urinary tract contaminations, and calm stomach exasperation. It has a comprehensive range of historical usages in diverse cultures, counting the dealing of diarrhea, arthritis, and various menstrual disorders. It is employed as an adjuvant in stomachic and carminative medicines and is also administered in cases of anorexia, inflammation, vomiting, and tubercular ulcers. It is very effective for rheumatism and inflammation, and its application in small quantities to the forehead gives relief in neuralgic headaches. It is also used externally as a rubefacient and is employed to counteract the stings of poisonous insects.

Bay Leaf

Botanical name: Laurus nobilis, Cinnamomum tamala

The origin of bay leaf is southern Asia, from where it spread to the rest of Asia and now all over the world. It is an aromatic leaf having a sharp, bitter taste, used in cooking mostly in dried form, either whole or powdered. The essential oil of bay leaves gives flavor and also extends the shelf life of foods because of its antimicrobial and antioxidant activities. Apart from essential oil, bay leaves have eugenol and flavonoids, which give antioxidant properties to bay leaves.

Medicinal uses: Bay leaf has many functional properties like antimicrobial and antifungal, hypoglycemic (in the control of diabetes), antiulcerogenic, antioxidant, and anti-inflammatory activity. The essential oil of bay leaf has a bactericidal action against many pathogens like

Staphylococcus aureus, Escherichia coli, Shigella flexnerii, and Salmonella typhi. Bay leaves are also useful for skin rashes, earache, and rheumatism.

Immunity Boosting Recipes

Recipe Example 1:

Ingredients:

- 1 teaspoon Cardamom powder

- 1 teaspoon Cinnamon powder

- 1 teaspoon dried ginger powder

- 1 teaspoon black pepper powder

- 2 tablespoons jaggery (optional)

- 400 ml water

Instructions:

1. In a big stainless-steel saucepan, add cardamom powder, cinnamon powder, dried ginger, powder, black pepper powder, and water. Boil the contents on low flame until the volume reduces to half. Add Jaggery and boil further till it dissolves. Drink it when the liquid is warm but not too hot.

2. This decoction is a drink of herbs and spices which are typically boiled in water for a length of time, allowing all of the medicinal benefits to be extracted. The formulation is especially useful in the cold and dry period when allergies can rise. When boiled, you can drink the decoction numerous times throughout the day. One can keep it and then warm just before drinking it. If you frequently become ill, it indicates that your body's immunity is near to the ground. You can reinforce it with the aid of this herbal drink, which has a mix of several

herbs. It will rouse digestion, upsurge immunity, and likewise detox your body. Black pepper and cardamom are suitable for flu and various allergic difficulties. Ginger and cinnamon also help digestion, which straightly influences our immunity, as our primary line of protection is in the gut.

Consume 50 ml daily once, after breakfast, for 3 weeks.

Recipe Example 2:

Ingredients:

- ½ teaspoon cardamom powder

- ½ teaspoon clove powder

- 1 teaspoon turmeric powder

- ¼ teaspoon nutmeg powder

- 500 ml milk

- Honey (optional to taste).

Instructions:

1. Simply place all the fixings into a small pan and wait for it to a light boil, whisking to combine fixings. Stir rarely until it starts to boil. Remove from heat and serve. Strain the milk if you want to have clear, smooth milk. Add honey if desired.

2. Turmeric latte has been widely used as a strong blood purifier and cleanser in traditional systems of medicine, especially in Indian Ayurveda. The occurrence of a wide variety of dynamic nutrients in this milk boosts the immune system. The antioxidants in turmeric help to cleanse the lymphatic system, enhancing blood purification.

Consume warm milk, 100 ml daily after breakfast and after dinner, before going to bed. The course is for 3 weeks.

Recipe Example 3:

Ingredients:

- ½ teaspoon coriander seeds

- ½ teaspoon anise powder

- ¼ teaspoon black pepper powder

- ¼ teaspoon Indian long pepper

- 1/8 teaspoon asafoetida

- 1 tablespoon granulated sugar

- ¼ teaspoon rock salt

- 400 ml water

Instructions:

1. Boil water. Add all the ingredients except salt and sugar, and boil further till the volume reduces to 200 ml. Add sugar and salt and boil further till sugar dissolves and the mixture thickens a little bit. This is an aromatic water fortified with sugar and salt. It is an herbal salt and electrolyte replenisher with a carminative effect.

Consume 50 ml daily after breakfast. The course is 2 weeks.

Recipe Example 4:

Ingredients:

- 4 inches turmeric root (fresh)

- 4 inches ginger (fresh)

- 1 whole lime

- 200 grams sugar

- 200 ml water

Instructions:

1. Finely chop ginger and turmeric into fine slices and grind them to make a paste.

2. Add this paste to water for 5-10 minutes.

3. Strain to remove the herb pieces.

4. Add sugar to clear juice and squeeze the juice of 1 lime into it.

5. Boil it further till sugar dissolves and the mixture thickens.

A combination of ginger, turmeric and lemon is a powerful anti-oxidant, and has anti-inflammatory properties that protect the body from various bacterial infections by boosting the immune system. The combination of these three ingredients acts on different parts of the body and brain and is known to be a natural healer. Turmeric contains curcumin, which is an established anti-cancer, anti-oxidant, and anti-inflammatory agent. Ginger enhances metabolism, relieves stress, and helps to maintain blood pressure and blood sugar levels. Lemons are one of the richest sources of vitamin C, bile stimulant, and detox agent.

Consume 1 teaspoon twice a day, for up to 2 weeks.

Chapter 11. Alkaline Herbs and Natural Remedies for Health Problems

Herbs, together with a conscientious lifestyle, have power. Here are the best ten Alkaline Herbs.

Irish Sea Moss

As a facial mask, you can use Irish Sea Moss Gel to your face, which leaves your skin feeling moisturized and smooth. Irish Sea Moss is a perfect source for vitamin supplementation since it includes more than 100 minerals that are important for the human body.

Burdock Root

One of the main herbal teas is Burdock Root. This contains all of the body's 102 minerals, but at low levels. We are really much drink this herbal tea as it serves like a "blood cleanser," cleanses your lymphatic system, and functions as a natural laxative as well. There's a really slight earthy flavor to burdock root that we enjoy.

Soursop Leaves

One of the favorite herbal teas is Soursop Leaves. Soursop is popularly recognized for its anti-cancer & anti-parasitic effects. Soursop leaves go well with ginger, and for a great taste and anti-inflammatory drink, it is normally brewed together.

Elderberry

When you've got a cold and just want to give the immunity the boost, elderberries are perfect. Elderberries always help push the immune system but beware of how much as too much you eat might render you nauseous. Elderberries are a perfect addition to brewing tea with other herbs and is also useful for producing cough medicine.

Black Walnut Hull Powder

With its antibacterial, antiviral & anti-parasitic effects, it is perfect. This powder is added to the smoothies, or you can turn it into a tea as an option.

Dandelion Root

If you really want anything that feels similar to coffee, the dandelion root is great. Put hemp milk & date sugar, and you've got a latte that helps the liver cleanse. Coffee is acidic, but we prescribe it to coffee drinkers every morning as it cleanses the liver, ensuring it gives the energy to you as well (if that's why you drink coffee). A great way to detox and begin the morning is Dandelion Root.

Sarsaparilla Root

It is the richest in iron and thus suitable for requiring it. With other spices, like burdock root/dandelion root, Sarsaparilla goes well.

Bladderwrack Powder

For thyroid problems, arthritis, artery hardening, stomach diseases, heartburn, blood cleaning, constipation, urinary tract problems, bronchitis, and anxiety, Bladderwrack is used. Genuinely, because of its tremendous minerals and its ability to help strengthen the immune system and improve efficiency, we use Bladderwrack material. Apply smoothies to this powder, and you can barely taste it. Bladderwrack powder is sometimes used on the skin. Bladderwrack is healthy for the skin and incorporates properties that are anti-aging.

Damiana

People like Damiana because when they feel mentally unbalanced or upset, it makes them feel comfortable. As a natural aphrodisiac, Damiana is often widely used. Both males and females can use Damiana. Damiana is also a fantastic herb for the ladies as they encounter their menses.

Chamomile Flower

Because of its relaxing and mentally stimulating effects, it is one of the favorite teas. As it deals with anxiety and is really calming, Chamomile is a perfect tea to drink a night. For those battling depression, anxiety, and tension, chamomile is a perfect treatment. Chamomile helped many to immensely relieve the depression and to make their sleep well at night.

Test each of these herbs to see which of them fits well for you. For one individual, what works may not actually work for another. It can be helpful to research and listen to someone about what to try but finding things out about yourself is the perfect way to learn what's right for you.

Natural Means to Solve Health Problems

Natural treatments for health are getting a significant moment right now on the wellbeing scene. Your store can be a fairly successful spot to locate health remedies, whether it's oil pulling to treat a myriad of problems or using apple cider vinegar to the face to clear up acne.

So, continue reading if you want to find out natural remedies to basic health problems. Right here, we've rounded up fifty of our picks.

- Bad breath: Try the oil pulling.

Try this if you feel like avoiding getting up near with individuals for fear of your bad breath, and flossing and brushing twice a day does little to improve. Oil pulling followers swear by the procedure's potential to freshen breath for even longer than a gum or an Altoid. Simply swish the coconut oil around a tbsp. for 20 mins per day before brushing your teeth.

- Cold & Flu: Dark Leafy Greens

Jessica Sepel, nutritionist & Instagram sensation, advises consuming dark, leafy greens & Vitamin C to reduce colds or flu: "I'm a true believer in the whole foods in providing immune protection. Dark, leafy greens always are my go-to."

Vitamin C is a favorite on my desk when to supplements it comes, and it targets the virus's nucleic acid, and it continues hitting the infection until it's gone. Many people use Vitamin C Whole Foods as it's made from beautiful sources of whole food such as Acerola Cherry, Amla Berry, and Camu Camu. They are more bio-available to the bodies, and they are whole foods, which potentially enhances their immune-boosting abilities.

- PMS: Try using Magnesium

For many women, Magnesium is crucial in alleviating PMS symptoms. "It helps ease and calm the muscle, which helps the cramps," Sepel says.

For a natural dosage of Magnesium, look at foods including sunflower seeds, almonds, and vegetables like broccoli and spinach.

- Indigestion: Use peppermint

To relieve digestive problems such as indigestion, gas, nausea, and cramps, peppermint, peppermint oil, and peppermint tea are important.

- Thin, fragile nails: Consider massaging your nails with coconut oil.

Ditch the chemicals for genuine coconut oil.

- Anxiety: Use meditation

If someone suffers from anxiety before they start taking drugs, this will pay off to pursue meditation, here's how. People with an elevated risk of cardiovascular disease, sleep disorders, weight gain, and concentration and memory decline have been related to persistent stress. Regular therapy has also been reported in research to better control the effects of depressive disorders, sleep disturbances, depression, cancer, and cardiac disease. Actually, meditation works, so you can try it.

- Dry, flaky skin: seek honey

Not only is it affordable in the beauty line than everything else, but honey also softens & moisturizes dry skin, and it can be directly applied to trouble areas.

- Headache: Give acupuncture a shot.

Since the beginnings of Conventional Chinese Medicine, acupuncture is used to alleviate headaches. A 2009 research found that acupuncture helps decrease the severity and frequency of frequent sufferers of headaches.

- Weight issues: Pursue healthy fat for weight problems

Sepel advises adding more healthier fats into the diet and eliminating something labeled as low-fat/fat-free if you have been gaining weight gradually, and it won't appear to budge.

Sugar is loaded with reduced-fat and fat-free, and the body absorbs excess sugar as fat. Don't forget about healthier fats such as avocado, nuts, olive oil, and seeds-they provide you a boost of energy and hold you full longer, and they're filled with fiber and vitamin B- that help purify the bloodstream to continue to enjoy vegetables. A healthy body is a lean body, "she added."

- Pain during periods: Use Vitamin D

Hot water bottles, stretching, and painkillers are all standard approaches to reduce period pain; however, here's something you definitely haven't heard about vitamin D. When they were offered an ultrahigh amount of vitamin D 5 days before their next anticipated cycle, a limited group of people who normally felt extreme menstrual cramps reported substantially reduced pain.

- Lower back Sore: Consider Pilates

Strengthening the abdominal muscles will significantly boost lower back pain by muscle-lengthening activities like Pilates.

- Eczema: Pursue baths of Magnesium

It is known that magnesium bath salts cure eczema.

- Headaches: Use the peppermint oil

For treating a headache, peppermint oil is also added to the skin. Peppermint oil may induce surface warmth as it is added to the skin, which relieves
discomfort under the skin.

- Stress: Avoid caffeine.

Caffeine raises adrenaline inside the body and may trigger discomfort, so if you feel tense, stop it.

- Sore muscles: Go for ice therapy

Although a warm bath can provide instant relief to exhausted, overworked muscles, icing with ice wrapped in a wet towel usually avoids more injury to the muscle and will speed up the recovery phase of the muscle.

- Joint pain or Arthritis: Consider Turmeric

Turmeric is a yellow herb that has been used for 2,000 years in Ayurvedic medicine in India and China. Anecdotal research suggests that it is beneficial in the treatment of soft tissue inflammation in cases of arthritis. Try turmeric tea, or while cooking, sprinkle it over the food.

- Infections of the urinary tract: consider starting liver detox cleanse.

Although the dosage of antibiotics recommended by the doctor can typically remove the urinary tract's inflammation, Sepel states that they may often be a symptom of candida, which could naturally be helped.
To wash away the system, we suggest a liver-detox cleanse. She said that my 'Restart Plan' is an easy, healthy, and really delicious way to cut some of the inflammatory, sugary foods that feed the yeast and relieve frequent UTIs.

- Hangover: Consider bananas and coconut water

Coconut water is a strong hydrator that is essential to drinking after a long night out and has 5 electrolytes that our bodies require: potassium, sodium, phosphorus, magnesium, and calcium. When you consume alcohol, the body still lacks potassium, and bananas will let you replenish it.

- Vertigo: Use basil

A common remedy for vertigo aromatherapy is Basil: To the boiling water, add the leaves, and aid with vertigo and breathe in the steam.

- Pimples: Use Apple cider vinegar

We enjoy having apple cider vinegar-it works wonders on blemishes. Only rub a bit on the area, and overnight you'll see progress, Sepel said.

- Cravings for Nicotine: Try exercising

Only quit smoking right now. Nice for you. Continue to work out every day for 30 mins — it has been proven to assist with cravings, which might help you quit the habit.

- Nausea: Use ginger

For curing nausea and diarrhea, ginger has been used for hundreds of years. For a perfect way to defeat nausea, add some minced, new ginger with lemon in hot water.

- Hiccups: Use apple cider vinegar

It has a number of applications, but it has been proven that the strong and sour taste helps get rid of hiccups.

- Anemic: Use green vegetables, liver, and red meat.

Low levels of energy. Maybe you would like to check the amounts of iron. It's essential for women to eat lots of iron, so make sure your consumption of leafy green vegetables & red meat is adequately high.

- Dry cuticles: use honey, olive oil, and aloe vera

In the cup, mix the raw honey, olive oil, and aloe vera juice, then use as a hand cream and rub the cuticles. Repeat this every week several times.

- Infections of the Urinary Tract: Use cranberry juice

Research indicates that the advantageous substances in the cranberry juice could enter the urinary tract to prevent bacterial adhesion inside 8 hours, according to Web MD. However, get to the hospital if recurrent are the UTIs.

Chapter 12. First Aid Using Herbal Medicine

Common First Aid

In addition to the usual bandages, adhesive plasters, cotton wool, lint, and scissors, the following will be found invaluable:

Antispasmodic tincture—for the relief of any type of nerve pain, taken in warm water, and also massaged over the painful area; to ease the effects of shock, for nausea and sickness; good as a quick tonic when feeling tired or
- dejected and for nervousness. *Comfrey oil*—to apply immediately to any bruises, sprains, or injuries, will
- relieve the pain very quickly. *Bach Rescue Remedy*—to counteract shock of any kind, can be taken every few
- minutes if necessary.

Distilled witch-hazel—a soothing, gentle astringent to apply to bruises, sprains, insect bites, painful varicose
- veins, burns and sunburn, and as a compress on the eyes; will arrest hemorrhage.

Tincture of myrrh—an antiseptic, to apply well-diluted to wounds, bites, etc. It will smart. Apply neat to mouth
- ulcers.

Composition essence—taken in hot water to counteract
- chills and a feeling of chilliness; useful also for diarrhea.

Elderflower, peppermint, and composition—will ward off incipient colds, flu, etc.; taken in hot water will
- promote perspiration.

Chamomile flowers—to relieve nausea and sickness in
- adults and children; to calm the nerves.

Peppermint tea—for indigestion, will also ease headaches and relieve mental fatigue; useful for students at exam time.

Olbas oil (or some other herbal liniment)—to rub the chest in chesty colds or bronchitis, like an inhaler; to rub aching muscles.

Chickweed ointment—to heal wounds, lacerations, etc.; for burns, wasp and bee stings, to draw abscesses.

Oil of lavender—to repel insects or to apply to insect stings; smoothed gently on the temples will ease migraine's headaches.

Slippery elm—a soothing drink for many digestives and bowel disorders; useful also as a poultice.

Marshmallow root—very often gives effective relief to cystitis sufferers.

Raspberry leaves or Agrimony herb—to gently control diarrhea in both adults and children.

Powdered ginger—to ease painful flatulence and indigestion, a half-teaspoonful in a little hot water to be sipped slowly.

Holiday First Aid

One would not wish to appear to be a hypochondriac by carrying a large bagful of remedies 'just in case', but a few well-chosen items could prevent a holiday from being ruined. These would be selected from the domestic first aid box and could well include:

Antispasmodic tincture—for nerve pains, shock, and stomach upsets; to take to relieve sunstroke.

Distilled witch-hazel—for sunburn, burns, bruises, and bleeding, insect bites.

- *Bach Rescue Remedy*—to counteract a shock, including sunstroke.

- *Composition essence*—in hot water for chills; in cold water to help control diarrhea.

- *Tincture of meadowsweet*—in conjunction with composition essence, will control stomach upsets and diarrhea. Can be given to children.

- *Oil of lavender*—to repel insects; to help relieve headaches.

- *Chamomile tea*—for nausea; to calm the nerves.

- *Peppermint tea*—to relieve indigestion; to ease headaches.

- *Olbas oil*—to rub aching muscles; to rub the chest in colds and coughs; to inhale.

Chapter 13. Herb Garden

Growing an Herb Garden

W beginning, you'll find that gardening is much more than simply growing plants. Growing your own garden can be one of the most fulfilling experiences possible.hetheryouhavealready discovered that you have a green thumb and a pension for growing plants that thrive under your care, or you are just

Growing your own garden is a great way to nurture a connection between you and nature. Tending and observing your own garden gives your insight into the cycles and rhythms of nature. One of the simplest joys can be found in watching as a tiny seed grows into a tiny sprout and then into maturity.

Growing an herb garden is a great way to create a connection between you and the earth. You can watch the natural cycles of nature and connect with the healing plants that it offers. You can also rest assured that your herbs are of the highest natural quality.

If you are worried about trying to grow an herb garden of your own, then fear not. Herbs are one of nature's hardiest plants and have a knack for growing in less than optimal conditions. Simply give them the right conditions: water, light, and soil, and they will thrive beyond your wildest dreams.

Not so long ago, it was common for nearly every household to have their own kitchen herb garden so that they could create herbal remedies. Many people still do this today, and you can too.

Designing Your Own Herb Garden

The design that you choose for your home garden depends on your personal preferences and needs. Herbs can do well growing alongside both vegetables and flowers. However, you can also create and design a garden that is devoted especially to herbs.

When you plant your herbs depends on what type you're growing; however, the best idea is to plant them the same way that you would vegetable seedlings. You should wait until all danger of frost is gone before planting them out in the garden. This actually works best for most herbs due to the fact that they are not overly cold-tolerant. This way, you get them in the ground under the best conditions: warm air, warm soil, and a nice summer ahead of them. This is the best way to encourage robust growth.

If you already have a garden and wish to simply incorporate herbs, then you have two options:

Herbs & Flowers

The best kinds of herbs to plant alongside flowers are the ones, which have flowers and blooms of their own, and the ones that can contribute to attractive foliage. A few favorite choices for planting alongside flowers include: borage, Artemisia, basil (the purple-leaved one especially), dill, mint, and sage (the ones with colorful leaves too).

Herbs & Vegetables

Incorporating edible herbs into your already existing vegetable garden is a great idea because they both like the same growing conditions, fertile soil, and full sunlight. The best part is that when you're in the mood for a delicious summer salad, you already have everything you need right there. Favorite choices for adding to the vegetable garden include: chives, fennel, thyme, cilantro, dill, parsley, and basil.

Many gardeners decided the best solution for their herb garden is simply to put them all in their own separate garden. If that is the case, then all you have to do is follow the usual rules for flower gardens. Taller herbs should be placed in the middle or to the back, and shorter ones in the front. This way, you can easily see and have access to everything.

Formal or Informal

There are many types of herb gardens to choose from, but in general, most of them can be boiled down to either formal or informal. If you are considering a formal garden, then you should plan ahead on paper. Create a geometric design and the layout. Then add the pathways and edgings. This includes gravel, rocks, bricks, and even grass. You could even use plants as edgings, such as a sheared low hedge of dusty miller or lavender, germander, or small boxwood plants.

If you are leaning more towards an informal herb garden, you should consider making a plan for it on paper as well. A casual little herb garden can either look delightfully disorganized or like a tangled mess. The best advice would be to set up the same way that you would a flower or vegetable garden. Afterward, you can see how it looks and make changes as you see fit.

Caring for Herbs

Caring for herbs is much like caring for any other perennial or annual; however, they may have a few special needs. Any plant has its own growing requirements, but for the most part, herbs are not high maintenance plants. Most will require full sunlight and fertile soil that is well-drained. This way, they get plenty of moisture without suffering from overwatering.

There are a few things that you can do to ensure that your chosen herb garden site meets these requirements. For starters, you can trim shrubs and overhanging trees to ensure that there is plenty of sunlight. If you are concerned about the soil, adding organic matter (dampened peat moss, compost, etc.) and some sand can help improve its texture and fertility.

You should know that herbs rarely need any fertilizer. In fact, it may actually inhibit the health of the plant. Excess fertilizer can inhibit flowering or lead to unattractive growth that is vulnerable to pests and diseases.

Some herbs prefer soil with a higher pH balance, alkaline soil, or "sweeter" soil. If your garden soil is more acidic, then sprinkling some lime powder or chips around the base of the herb during planting time can fix this. Some herbs like this are lavender, Chia, and Echinacea.

One of the most important things to remember is to water your herb plants on the day you plant them, as well as in the following weeks ahead. This helps you ensure that you are getting them off to a good start. Once they are well-established, they are more likely to be somewhat drought tolerant.

There are also some herbs that prefer the soggy ground. However, the drawback to putting them in the soggy ground is that they may grow like wildfire. So, you should be willing to let them grow as they wish. If you live somewhere where that is not such a practical idea, then simply raise them in a pot and keep them well watered. You could also set the pot in a saucer of water so that the soil will continually stay a team. A few herbs that are like this include: Sorrell, golden seal, cardamom, chervil, bee balm, and mints.

Another great thing about growing herbs is that they are fun and easy to grow indoors, which also tends to extend the harvest time is cold winters are an issue. They grow best when they are on a windowsill where they can get plenty of sun. A kitchen windowsill is preferable so that they are handy when you need to use them for a recipe. Also, they add a pleasant fragrance and character to your kitchen.

As potted plants incline to grow towards their basis of sunlight, they can often begin to face or look one-sided. The way to avoid this is to put them a quarter turn occasionally so that they'll look healthier, fuller, and more balanced.

As a new herb gardener, you may be reluctant to trim or harvest too often. Unfortunately, this is a major mistake that many new herb gardeners make. Most herbs are very confined when grown in pots, so it is best to harvest or trimmed them often. If this is not done, then they may start to look sloppy or lanky. Trimming encourages them to grow more thickly and neatly, as well as to branch.

One of the things about herbs is this: they may eventually, naturally peter out and then will have to be replaced. So be sure to enjoy them to the fullest extent while they are in their prime.

Chapter 14. Herbs for Mental Health and Function

I scientifically proven to work effectively to make you very productive and healthy. Choosing from a number of these suggested herbs can really make a difference.nordertomaintain a sharp, healthy as well as an alert mind, you need to use a number of natural herbs that do not have side effects. These herbs are

Ginseng

This herb has been found to improve memory and mental performance while offering other benefits such as stimulation of the immune system and lowering of blood cholesterol. Ginseng is also effective in treating problems such as anxiety as well as improving resistance to stress and depression. Men and women taking ginseng herb have shown more ability to withstand stress and depression.

Ginseng root contains panaxosides or ginsenosides, active ingredients that are responsible for the medicinal properties. The herb is suitable for you in fighting fatigue, effects of stress, cholesterol levels, and preventing infections. Having good mental health contributes to the anti-aging effect, and ginseng has the ability to reduce degeneration of the blood stream, as well as improving mental performance.

Kudzu

Kudzu herb, also known as Japanese arrowroot, is recommendable, especially if you want to improve your drinking habits and reduce the killing of brain cells. The herb functions by regulating the drinking of alcohol through communication to the brain, alerting it that a certain amount is sufficient. Taking this herb will thus ensure that you don't end up drinking too much alcohol. Actually, a 7 day's treatment with an extract of the kudzu vine reduces alcohol consumption in binge drinkers. Kudzu's active ingredients, such as puerarin, are also effective in increasing blood flow to the brain and heart, particularly in emergencies.

Chamomile

This herb is effective in dealing with stress as well as calming the nerves and relieving menstrual cramps. You can use chamomile in herbal tea form or as a topical cream, with oral dosage recommendable being 9 -15 grams daily. Chamomile oil contains a-bisabolol as oxides, spiro-ether or farnesene, which possesses anti-inflammatory and antispasmodic properties.

An effective way of taking the herb is incorporating it in tea or another beverage so as to reduce tension and maintain your brain health. Drinking a warm concoction is the best natural way for a soothing effect.

Holy Basil

Holy basil is also known as tulsi and is effective in reducing stress by hindering the build-up of cortisol. This herb can also improve cerebral circulation and memory while at the same time relieving cloudy thinking and general mental fog. Holy basil can also treat attention deficit disorder, attention deficit hyperactivity disorder, and other forms of depression. Holy basil leaf extract contains a synergistic effect with silymarin, the active ingredient that is made of various flavonoids.

Bacopa

Bacopa originates from India and has been confirmed to be effective in improving memory, learning, and cognition response. You can take the herb to improve your old memories as it contains active ingredients such as triterpene glycosides. This substance enhances the efficiency in the transmission of nerve impulses. Bacopa also contains antioxidant properties, which offer protection against brain damage.

Taking a bacopa liquid herbal extract will provide you with benefits such as improved cognitive function, focus, and emotional wellbeing.

Valerian

Lack of sleep can be effectively treated with naturally occurring valerian herb that functions better than traditional sleeping pills and eliminates side effects. Valerian herb contains isovalerate, an active ingredient known for its medicinal properties. Using the herb will relieve you from problems such as insomnia, sleeplessness, and restless nights, as valerian root has a sedative and soothing impact.

Valerian root is recommendable as it does not cause sleepiness or drowsiness during the daytime. The root also acts as a muscle relaxant and can be used to effectively reduce muscle cramps and spasms.

Chapter 15. Herbs for Everyday Use

Many of them promise to be the best for your health. But whether you are growing these herbs in a garden or purchasing them online, you are not able to keep hundreds of herbs in your home just in case you need them. henyou aregetting startedonusing herbal remedies,youmaybe confused about where to begin. There are hundreds of different herbs to use, and

One of the first things that people will ask when they get started with herbs is which herbs they should keep on hand. Here is a list of the top herbs that you should consider having on hand as you begin your journey with herbal remedies.

Over time, you will learn which herbs you like and which ones work out the best with your needs and the needs of your family, but these are good ones to get started with.

Echinacea

This is one of the best herbs to have around when winter time comes. It is good for helping out with sore throats, the flu, and colds during the winter as well as some of the other respiratory infections you may be dealing with. Echinacea works so well with these conditions because it works to boost up the immune system and is a strong antibiotic. Keeping a bit on hand and using it during the flu and cold season can make a big difference in your health.

Garlic

While you may already be using garlic in your regular cooking, there are so many other great uses that come from adding garlic into your diet. First off, garlic is good at reducing your blood pressure and your cholesterol levels, making it a great herb to take when you need to help out that heart. It also fights off infections and boosts your immunity, so you are less likely to get sick.

To help out your heart and to lower your risk of infections, it is best to consume some garlic on a daily basis. If you like to add some flavoring to your cooking, adding a bit of garlic to a meal will often do the trick and give you the benefits.

If you aren't a big fan of the taste of garlic, consider getting a supplement or a capsule with garlic inside so that you can take care of your heart.

Chamomile

If you are someone who loves to have some tea before going to bed, you are probably a big fan of chamomile. This is often seen as the pleasure herb, but it is used more as a remedy to help reduce stress and help you to relax. If you are dealing with a lot of stress from work or you have issues with insomnia, chamomile is one of the first things that many people will suggest to make these issues easier to handle.

In addition to helping you to fall asleep and reduce the amount of stress that is in your life, chamomile will work to solve many other issues, including stuffy nose and indigestion. Just having a cup or two of tea with some chamomile on a daily basis can help you out so much with these common issues.

Hawthorn

For those who are dealing with heart disease or have a family history of heart disease, hawthorn should be one of the herbs that are in your medicine cabinet. It is one of the best herbs to use when it comes to protecting your heart and can be used in an extract form to keep that heart strong. Take hawthorn as a preventative method before heart issues occur or any time that you feel that your heart needs a little added bonus.

Aloe Vera

This is one that you may already have inside of your home. Aloe Vera is the main ingredient found in most products that are used to treat burns, whether it is a burn from a fire or from the sun. Keeping some of this on hand can give you a bit of relief after a long day in the sun or if you get a nasty burn that just won't feel relief any other way.

In addition to helping you with your burns, Aloe Vera can work nicely to help out with bites and burns. If you use the juice from their herb, it is great at

helping out with your upset stomachs. If possible, growing Aloe Vera in your home is the best option because you will be able to grab the fresh leaves

right when you need them for the best results. Of course, any type of Aloe Vera will work nicely, and you will get the relief that you need even if it is not fresh.

Eucalyptus

Another herb that you may want to consider for your medicine cabinet is eucalyptus. This one has a unique smell that a lot of people like to have on hand, and it is perfect for clearing out a stuffy nose or chest. In fact, this herb is one of the main ingredients that are found in many cold remedies, including Vick's Vapor Rub, because it does such a good job at clearing out the sinuses. Having this inside an herbal steam or in a hot cup of tea can make you feel better as well.

There are many uses of eucalyptus for your overall health. It is good for helping out with a head or chest cold, sinusitis, stuffy nose, and a cough. It can also help to keep you calm and release some of the feelings of anxiety that you may be feeling throughout your day. Consider keeping some eucalyptus on hand for those colds, and you will feel better in no time.

Ginger

Ginger is one of the best herbs to use when you are trying to fight off inflammation in the body. This makes it good for all kinds of arthritis that could be affecting how great you feel through the day. Not only is ginger good for helping prevent inflammation, but it can help with motion sickness, nausea, and chest congestion.

Many times, pregnant women are prescribed some ginger, such as ginger ale, to help out when they are dealing with morning sickness.

Ginger is available in many different forms. You can get the root in powdered form and use this inside of drinks, teas, and even your food. Other options are in capsules and other supplements so you can get all the great benefits.

Peppermint

You just can't go wrong with having some peppermint in your home when you get started with herbal remedies. Not only does it smell amazing, but it is able to help out so much with the different aspects of your health. First off, if you are dealing with an upset stomach, peppermint is really good at helping to ease these pains and make you feel better. If you add it in with some honey and chamomile, it can work to ease even the delicate stomach of a young child. Many families like peppermint because it is gentle enough for even their children to use.

If you add in peppermint to some lemon juice, it can help to soothe your sore throat, and it is often used to help out with other cold symptoms because it is a good decongestant. Many people have used peppermint or spearmint as well to help them lose weight because it is believed that peppermint can help to suppress the appetite.

Lavender

Lavender is a perfect herb to keep on hand for anyone who is suffering from stress, anxiety, depression, and even having trouble with sleeping. Lavender works well to handle all of these issues, no matter how big or small they may seem. If the stress at work is getting you down or you feel down because things don't seem to go your way, drink a bit of lavender tea at the end of the day. If you are someone who has trouble getting to sleep on a regular basis and suffers from insomnia, just get a little infuser and mix in the lavender oil as you slowly fall into a deep sleep. It is gentle and calming for anyone to use, and you will be amazed at how much better you feel when you use it.

Rosemary

Rosemary has been around for many years and is good for those who need help with their memory. Whether you are just having trouble keeping the focus that you need to get through the day or you are dealing with the early signs of dementia, rosemary could be the herb that you need to feel better. This one also works well in many different kinds of foods, so you can easily add them to your meals to get all the great benefits.

As you can see, there are many different types of herbs that you can use in your life. These are just a few of the most popular options that you can keep on hand in case you need an uplift, help with burns and cuts, or something else that goes on in your daily life. Consider keeping some of these on hand or adding them to your collection to ensure that you are set for all of the situations that come up in your life.

Chapter 16. Natural Remedies for the Digestive Problems

I However, do keep in mind *to practice herbal and natural remedies with caution*. Even something that is "of the Earth" can have dangers, especially if a person has an allergy/sensitivity to a certain ingredient.t'stimetodivein and learnabout some of the proven techniques to rid oneself of stomach ailments—without the nasty side-effects of regular drugs.

Bloat/Gas

Activated Charcoal

Although it's scientifically inconclusive exactly why charcoal is so beneficial to the stomach, it's known to help a variety of gastro problems, including gas. The type to buy is "activated" charcoal, where it's oxidized usually by a process of steaming. The steam punches tiny holes through the charcoal, which makes it become porous. Much as we use charcoal as a natural filter for purifying water, these pores will also trap toxins in your body and may absorb the pathogens leading to your gastro ailments.

Apple Cider Vinegar

Vinegar is another ancient and trusted remedy. Firstly, it helps to balance our pH levels with its strong alkaline properties, and secondly, it works as an internal cleanser. If you are experiencing gas, try adding 2 tbsp. of apple cider vinegar to a glass of warm water.

Asafoetida

This middle-eastern herb, similar to leeks, is another ancient stomach remedy that is commonly served in or with meals from India, Iran, Pakistan, Afghanistan, and many other countries. Specifically, it is known as an anti-flatulent and directly helps to cure gas and bloat.

To obtain the herb, it's best to order it. It usually comes bottled and powdered, and it can be added as a tasteful seasoning to various dishes. However, if you can find the herb whole (again, at a good import supermarket), this might be your best bet to immediately relieve gas. In this form, it's commonly eaten raw as part of Middle Eastern salad dishes. The taste and aroma have been known to be a bit strong to first-time eaters.

Baking Soda and Lemon

This mixture naturally forms carbon dioxide, which can equalize your digestive tract during a bout of gas and is a very effective remedy.

Fill up one glass of water and add 2 tbsp. of lemon juice and 1 ½ teaspoon of baking soda. Stir with a spoon, and watch as it begins to fizz. After the fizz has lessened, drink the tonic.

Fennel

As with asafetida, fennel is another herb indigenous to the Middle East and many parts of the Mediterranean coast. It is a spicy, aromatic herb that is prepared in many dishes on that side of the world. Fennel seeds are even used in many Italian recipes, like in sausages and cured meats.

Aside from being a bountiful ingredient, fennel is famous for digestive assistance and, in particular—curing gas. Eat a serving of dried fennel seeds (with adequate chewing). Many reports that after doing this, gas is immediately expelled from where it may be lodged in the intestines.

Fennel seeds have some side effects, especially among sufferers of epilepsy, so research whether fennel is right for you before consuming any.

Ginger

This root is famous for its digestive properties and has been used for these purposes for thousands of years. In terms of curing gas/bloating, it's very effective.

The best type of ginger, in my opinion, is called Gari, which is a Japanese thinly sliced salmon-pink colored young ginger. This is commonly found alongside most meals at Japanese restaurants, and it may be available pre-sliced at certain foreign grocery stores.

Eat 9-10 pieces, chewing thoroughly.

Ground Turmeric

According to studies by the University of Maryland medical center, the spice turmeric holds multiple benefits for the digestive tract, including stimulating the gallbladder to produce bile.

Turmeric is usually purchased in powdered form. From there, it has many recipes and uses. You can try adding 2 tsp. to a full glass of milk (creating a golden effect and a tasty flavor). Or, you can find it as an ingredient in many spicy mustards. Mustard has other health benefits as well, which may further help your digestion. Try eating two full tablespoons of the mustard by itself.

Turmeric can be found in many healthy foods, or it <u>can also be ordered online</u>.

Probiotic Cocktails

Before you've heard me mention the importance of probiotics for digestive health. What many don't realize is that there are many more options besides
just yogurts, and they can provide relatively quick stomach relief for gas sufferers. Try:

- One half cup Sauerkraut

- 1-2 servings of Kimchee (Korean fermented cabbage dish. Available at foreign grocers and Korean restaurants.)

- 2-3 whole pickles

- 1 bottle of Kefir (sour fermented milk drink)

- 1 cup of buttermilk

- Or 1-2 servings of probiotic yogurt.

Spearmint / Peppermint Tea or Essence of Mint

Menthol, the active ingredient of mint, is famous for its anti-nausea properties. In addition, mint-o-philes claim that it can even be a quick-fix for bouts of gas and other abdominal upsets.

Find a pure form of peppermint tea bags, and prepare the tea by steeping it in boiled water, covered, for approx. 15 minutes to make a strong cup. Add a touch of sweetener (preferably honey) and sip.

Stress

Not to sound like a broken record, as I mentioned the factors of stress and indigestion before. But what are some specific actions you can take to immediately lower this negative emotion in your life?

First of all, I think a lot of times stress can be eliminated. My brother suffered from a bad ulcer during a very (unnecessarily, I might add) stressful point in his life. However, much of his worrying could have been alleviated (as well as his doctor bills) had he taken some steps to relax.

I could write another book about stress relief—but I think the best way to solve stress is to solve your problems, so you don't have to worry about them.

It might be the stack of bills on the counter or a hard conversation with someone that you've been putting off.

Meditation works, but if you have unfinished business on your mind, I think it's very hard to relax enough to even meditate.

Personally, if I know I have something that needs to get taken care of and I haven't done it, no amount of soothing music or other techniques is going to help.

So, figure out what your problems are, compile them, and then start knocking them out of your mind! When everything's done, you'll find it becomes much easier to relax.

And then, when you're able to relax enough with immediate pressures out of your mind, I'd suggest to start meditation practices. I talk about these types of concepts more thoroughly in other books.

Increase Acid Levels

It may sound odd, but doctors have found that acid reflux is often the result of not having enough acid, not because you have too much. The lower esophageal sphincter tightens when the acid levels deplete, and that tightness sends the remaining acid up your digestive tract.

Some ways to increase acidity include:

- The juice of 1/3rd a lemon squeezed into a glass of water with a bit of sweetener (a strong lemonade)

- Sea salt

- Apple cider vinegar

- Some servings of acidic fruit.

For the salt, your best option is the unprocessed kind (Himalayan), and this is probably the best remedy of all for equalizing your acidic levels. This is because chloride is used by the body to produce (hydro) chloric acid, which is the chemical that you use to digest food. The salt replenishes this chemical in a raw form.

Try sprinkling it in earnest on some vegetables, like steamed cabbage.

As for fruit, try it as a last resort because acidic fruit is sometimes hard to digest and may make symptoms worse.

Finally, please note that lemons and vinegar have an unusual property where they are both acidic and alkaline (I'll talk more about this in a minute). Many health professionals agree it's better for your body to remain alkaline in nature, fortunately counteracting a pH imbalance is not the same as acidifying your body, and these foods will actually increase your overall alkalinity levels.

Ginger Again?

As mentioned before, ginger works digestive miracles. In addition to trying the sliced pink Japanese ginger, I'd suggest buying some ginger root tea.

If you buy the tea from a retailer, avoid a powdered or leafy "herbal" tea. You want to buy sliced or diced fresh ginger that can be steeped as you would a regular teabag.

Many health food stores provide ginger in this form. Allow the tea too steep for 20 minutes, and put the batch in the fridge to warm up anytime you begin to experience indigestion symptoms.

Wean Off Medications

OK. Many medications cause heartburn and indigestion, and patients don't even know it. These effects can be even worse if combined with a poor diet or if the medication is taken without enough food in your stomach.
Some drugs that cause indigestion as a side effect include:

- Antidepressants

- Anti-anxiety

- Blood pressure

- Antibiotics.

Obviously, don't go cold turkey on your meds. Instead, talk to your doctor about your indigestion problems, and seek out a timeline for when you can stop taking the drugs.

In this day and age, I see so many who get on anti-anxiety or anti-depressant drugs and never finish their need for them. The idea behind these drugs is for patients to take them for as long as they suffer from the problem. And then, through psychiatric therapy, they don't have to use them anymore.

But instead, people keep taking the same drugs for years and years, and all of the nasty side-effects that go with them.

If you suffer from indigestion or other issues because of such medications, please think about working with your doctor to create a strategy where you don't have to keep taking them forever.

Alkalinity

Just like acid may actually equalize your acidic levels, it is ALSO possible to treat reflux with alkalinity. This is because the alkaline properties will neutralize the acid in your esophagus (although it may not necessarily stop the *cause* of the reflux).

There are different ways to get a nice shot of alkalinity:

- Mustard

As with other remedies, a spoonful of Dijon mustard is a nice alkaline booster.

- Peppers

Most peppers are alkaline in nature. While hot peppers might hurt your gastrointestinal tract, some mild yellow peppers should be fine (like the kind we eat on hot-dogs or hoagies). Eat a nice serving with crackers.

- Apple Cider Vinegar

Again, with the vinegar! Now, you may be a little bit confused, as vinegar was just listed as an acidic remedy, right?

As I mentioned earlier, despite the fact that vinegar is acidic, it actually has an alkaline effect on our bodies! Don't ask me to explain the chemical reasons behind this, as it's way over my head.

Chapter 17. Natural Remedies for the Respiratory Ailments

Hyssop Oxymel

Indications:

Take this homemade hyssop oxymel by the teaspoonfuls throughout the day to treat coughs and congestion.

Ingredients:

- 1 cup Honey, raw

- A large handful hyssop, dried

- 2 cups of apple cider vinegar

Instructions:

1. Chop the dried hyssop herb into small bits. Place inside a glass jar.

2. Pour the raw honey into the jar, making sure the dried hyssop bits are completely covered.

3. Top the honey-hyssop mixture with the apple cider vinegar.

4. After labeling the jar, let stand for two weeks to one month.

5. Strain the mixture through a clean cheesecloth.

6. Transfer the hyssop oxymel in a clean airtight bottle, label, and store in a cool, dry place.

Herbal Cough Drops

Indications:

These herbal cough drops work effectively in taming those dry coughs at night.

Ingredients:

- Sage leaves, dried (1 tablespoon)

- Hyssop leaves, dried (1 tablespoon)

- Thyme leaves, dried (1 tablespoon)

- Sugar, organic (2 cups)

- Blackstrap molasses, organic (3/4 cups)

- Water (1 cup)

- Rose petal powder (1 tablespoon)

Directions:

1. Use a bit of melted coconut oil to grease a casserole dish or cookie sheet. Set aside.

2. Pour the water into a medium bowl. Add the dried hyssop, thyme, and sage leaves and stir to combine.

3. Cover the bowl and allow the mixture too steep for about fifteen minutes.

4. After straining off the dried herbs, take half a cup of the prepared tea.

5. Pour the strong herbal tea in a large saucepan. Add the organic sugar and blackstrap molasses, then stir well to combine.

6. Attach your candy thermometer to one side of the saucepan before heating on medium-high for fifteen minutes or until its temperature reaches 300 degrees.

7. Stir the mixture continuously so it does not burn. Take a spoonful of the mixture and drop into a bowl filled with cold water. If it instantly solidifies, then it is done.

8. Pour the mixture onto your greased casserole dish or cookie sheet.

9. Use one end of a rubber spatula to cut the semi-solid mixture into squares right away.

10. Dust the herbal cough drops with rose petal powder to prevent them from sticking to one another.

11. Store the herbal cough drops in an airtight jar and place in a cool, dry area.

Chamomile Herbal Steam (For Stuffy Nose)

Indications:

Relieving a stuffy nose is not a problem with this effective stuffy nose remedy. (You may reuse this chamomile tea several times, after which you can use it in your garden for composting.)

Ingredients:

- Chamomile flowers, dried (2 handfuls)

- Water (2 quarts)

Directions:

1. Pour the water into a pot and heat on medium-high. Allow the water to boil before turning off the heat and adding the dried chamomile flowers.

2. Cover the pot and allow the mixture to boil for an additional fifteen minutes.

3. Remove the pot from the heat and let stand on a large hot pad.

4. With plenty of tissues as well as a large towel on hand, remove the pot cover.

5. Holding your face over the steaming pot, place the towel on top of your head. Breathe in through the nose and mouth to let the steam unclog your stuffy nose (use the tissues to wipe your nose). Do this for five to fifteen minutes or until your stuffy nose is relieved.

Herbal Colds and Flu Tincture

Indications:

This spicy tincture has antibiotic and antiseptic properties that make it effective as a colds and flu herbal remedy. Take 1 teaspoon per hour when the colds and flu act up.

Ingredients:

- Vinegar (1 cup)

- Horseradish, fresh, grated (1 ½ tablespoons)

- Ginger, fresh, grated (1 ½ tablespoons)

- Onion, minced (1 ½ tablespoons)

- Garlic, minced (1 ½ tablespoons)

- Honey (1/3 cup)

- Mustard seeds (1 ½ tablespoons)

- Black peppercorns (1 ½ tablespoons)

- Cayenne chilies, whole (1 to 2 pieces) or chili flakes, dried (1 teaspoon)

Directions:

1. Take a glass jar (1 pint) and fill with the minced garlic and onion.

2. Add the grated horseradish and ginger along with the peppercorns, whole cayenne chilies or dried chili flakes, and mustard seeds. Stir well to combine.

3. Top the mixture with the vinegar, making sure there is an inch of liquid above the rest of the ingredients.

4. Cover with a lid made of plastic material. Allow the mixture to sit for two weeks, shaking the jar every day to ensure that the liquid and herbs are mixed.

5. Use a clean cheesecloth to strain the mixture.

6. Add the honey into the mixture before pouring into a clean, labeled bottle and storing in the cupboard.

Bee Balm Bronchial Oxymel

Indications:

Use this homemade bee balm oxymel to treat colds, flu, sore throats, and congested coughs.

Ingredients:

- Bee balm, fresh (enough to fill a whole glass jar)

- Apple cider vinegar, organic (enough to fill half of the jar)

- Honey, raw (enough to fill half of the jar)

Directions:

1. Fill an entire glass jar with the fresh bee balm.

2. Pour in the honey as well as the vinegar. Stir well to combine.

3. Cover the jar with a plastic lid (otherwise, line a metal lid with wax paper to protect the oxymel from contamination due to metal corrosion).

4. Allow the mixture to sit for a minimum of two weeks, stirring it from time to time to ensure that all ingredients are mixed well. (You might also try shaking the jar every so often.

5. Once the herbs are completely infused in the honey and vinegar, strain the mixture through several layers of clean cheesecloth. You may wring out the cheesecloths to get all that oxymel out, then discard the used herbs.

Marshmallow Root Pastilles

Indications:

These cooling, soothing marshmallow root pastilles work effectively in treating sore throats as well as heartburn, ulcers, and other digestive problems.

Ingredients:

- Rose petals, powdered (1 tablespoon)

- Sage leaves, powdered (1/2 tablespoon)

- Marshmallow root (2 tablespoons)

- Honey, raw, warmed (1 ½ tablespoons)

- Cinnamon powder (1/2 tablespoon)

  Rose powder (1/2 tablespoon)

-

Directions:

1. Combine the marshmallow root with the powdered rose petals and sage leaves in a mixing bowl.

2. Meanwhile, warm the honey in a small saucepan heated on medium. Make sure it never gets too hot, but just warm enough to have the consistency of a syrup.

3. Once the honey is warm, pour into the herb mixture in small amounts, stirring as you go. Keep stirring until you end up with a soft dough that is just sticky enough.

4. Use your clean hands to mold the pastille dough into small balls.

5. Sprinkle cinnamon and rose petal powders on the prepared pastilles before using immediately or storing in the refrigerator for about two weeks.

Conclusion

From the early days of humankind, plants, herbs, & ethnobotanicals have been used and are now being used worldwide for health promotion and disease care. In today's modern Medicine, plants and natural sources shape the foundation and contribute primarily to the industrial drug formulations developed today. About 25 percent of prescription medications globally are produced from plants. Even medicines are sometimes used in health treatment rather than medications.

Herbal therapy is, for others, their favorite therapeutic form. Herbs are used as an adjunct treatment to traditional pharmaceuticals, among others. In several emerging societies, moreover, conventional Medicine, to which herbal Medicine is a central component, is the only accessible or accessible health care method. Those utilizing herbal remedies should be confident, irrespective of the cause, that the items they are purchasing are healthy and contain what they are meant to contain, whether it be a single herb or a certain quantity of a single herbal ingredient. Science-based details on dose, contraindications, and effectiveness should also be provided to customers. Global harmonization of laws is required to accomplish this in order to direct the responsible development and selling of herbal medicines. If ample clinical proof of an herb's usefulness is present, that law may allow it to be used properly to encourage the utilization of that herb, such that those benefits may be appreciated for the protection of public health & the diagnosis of illnesses.

You've reached the end of the book, but not the end of your journey to using herbal medicine. I hope you've enjoyed what you've learned so far. As you start to practice and use herbal remedies, take some time to reflect on how well they work for you. A great way of doing this is by keeping a journal with the remedy that you used, the recipe you followed, and whether it worked or not. You can also include any side effects you had or any allergic reactions, so you know which remedies aren't for you. To maintain the safety and effectiveness of your herbal remedies, it's important to store them correctly. For infusions, you can store them in a covered jar in the fridge for 24 hours.

Herbal medicine is a safe, effective way to treat most illnesses. The key way to treat properly is to first understand what you are treating and choose a remedy that will work for that illness. Make sure the herbs you choose are correct and aren't misidentified or of poor quality. When you first purchase your herbs, remember to check them. Look at their color, shape, and fragrance. You want to make sure the herbs match what you're expecting and don't have any extras that don't match.

In the end, one must be thankful to the Native Americans for their role and task in providing us the benefits and usage of these natural remedies through herbs and plants. Nature is always kind to us, so we should be comfortable while using these herbs, and if you are reading this part of the book, you must be well informed about the uses, benefits, and side effects of herbal medicine and remedies.

CPSIA information can be obtained
at www.ICGtesting.com
Printed in the USA
LVHW050531160621
690357LV00007B/972

9 781802 431056